INSIDE-OUT

WEALTH

Holistic Wealth Creation

L. Michael Hall, Ph.D.

> Title Page

© 2010 **Inside-Out Wealth: Holistic Wealth Creation**
    A Neuro-Semantic Model for Creating Wealth
    L. Michael Hall, Ph.D.
    Copyright pending in Washington DC.

All Rights Reserved.
    No part of this may be reproduced, stored in a retrieval system, or transmitted in any form or by any means (electronic, mechanical, photocopying, recording, etc.) Without the prior *written permission* of the publisher.

ISBN: 978-1890001377

L. Michael Hall, Ph.D.
ISNS — *International Society of Neuro-Semantics®*
P.O. Box 8
Clifton, CO   81520
    (970) 523-7877

Web Sites:
    www.neurosemantics.com
    www.neuro-semantics-trainings.com
    www.meta-coaching.org
    www.self-actualizing.org

Audio and Video Recordings: There are audio and video recordings of the Wealth Creation training that Tom Welch has created. For more about that see the website: www.nlp-video.com.

Thanks to *Sue Anderson* (Australia) and *Brand Coetzee* (South Africa), both Meta-Coaches, for proof-reading the manuscript. *And* only hold me responsible for mis-spellings and grammatical mistakes. That's because after all of the work they devoted in making corrections, I transgressed the Law of Proof-Reading and made more changes, thereby ensuring additional mistakes. What to do? Ah, solution! I offer them to every perfectionist who reads this text for accuracy of typing and grammar rather than building a life of wealth!

INSIDE-OUT WEALTH

Preface   1

PART I: THE DREAM
1: Can Wealth be Created?   7
    Modeling Wealth Creation
2: How Long will it Take?   27
    The 7 stages of Wealth Creation
3: Why do it?   42
    Your Intentional Stance for an informed Decision
4: What are the Highest Meanings?   58
    The Heart of Wealth
5: What are the Best Meanings?   74

PART II: THE CORE   92
6: How do I get Started?   93
7: How can *I* create Wealth?   115
    Finding Your Singularity
8: Am I a Wealth Creator?   132
9: Who will go with me?   150
    Wealth Collaboration
10: Can I Make a Business Out of This?   166
    Entrepreneur-ing to see and seize Opportunities

PART III: THE STATES
11: What are the Best states?   183
12: What are the Highest States?   184
13: Can I have Fun Doing this?   213
14: What are the Principles of Wealth Creation?   222
    Mind-to-Muscle pattern
15: Your Wealth Creation Plan   235
    Your Ten-Year Plan

Appendices:
A: Time-binding Wealth   244
B: Wealth Creation Paradoxes   248
C: Mental Accounting   253
D: Millionaire Mind Checklist   256

Bibliography   263
Index   267
Author   270

PREFACE

*"What lies behind us and what lies before us are tiny matters
compared to what lies within us."*
Ralph Waldo Emerson

Everybody ought to be rich! And nearly everybody can be rich. I believe that and that's why I have written this book. Why do I believe these things about wealth? Because, typically, when a person has financial independence,[1] he or she can then focus on things other than money.

Paradoxical, isn't it? When money isn't dominating your every thought, you can focus on your gifts, your potentials, your best way of living, your best way of contributing to others, creating the best version of you, and the richest meanings and values of your life. *Then you can become truly wealthy in every dimension.*

True wealth is inside-out wealth. It does not come from the outside, it comes from the inside. When it does, then it is almost inevitable that you will also become wealthy on the outside in terms of finances, possessions, resources, opportunities, and a legacy of contribution.

While there are several secrets in wealth creation, this first one is the central one. *Wealth is an inside-out phenomenon.* This means several things of supreme importance for you.

It first means that to create wealth you have to begin by looking within to find your inner wealth—the inner wealth of your creative thoughts, abundant heart, and ability to create value for yourself and others. It then means that *you have tremendous wealth creation potentials—potentials that you can unleash.* And you begin to do that by actualizing your best competencies.

There are also several myths about getting wealthy. The key myth that will attempt to hijack your thoughts and feelings is the "Get Rich Quick" myth. Actually, the get-rich-quick mentality is a fast way to become poor, victimized, and deceived. It is the fastest way to become a sucker for a thousand schemes and to become deaf and blind to all of the possibilities around you for actually creating lasting wealth.

Conversely, the actual secret of wealth creation regarding time is that wealth creation requires long-term thinking. It is created by working through the stages of wealth creation with persistence, dedication, commitment, and discipline.

Models and Modeling
I created the *Inside-Out Wealth Creation* program described in this book by modeling wealth creators. I examined what they did behaviorally that created wealth; I explored their beliefs, values, states, meta-states, perceptual filters, and attitudes. Along the way I found numerous strategies for creating financial wealth that worked in the short-term, yet they were unhealthy strategies. Use them and you will pay a high price for money—for some of the people I modeled, it cost their health, for others their relationships, for others, their sanity and enjoyment of life.

The process for actually creating wealth is not rocket science. Learning and discovering how to do it is fairly simple. *Following through and actually doing it*—that's where it becomes tough. And that is where most people fail. So, the strategy is simple; the execution is not. For effective execution that actually implements the strategy you will need *inside-out mental frames of mind*—the mind of a Wealth Creator. That's what this book is about: identifying and integrating those mental frames.

After the creation of a model, a model that works, that maps out a legitimate, practical, and do-able strategy, then you need, as I did, a way to actually take on and integrate the model into your life and activities. A model that you cannot use for replicating the process in your life situation isn't worth the paper it's written on. That's where most wealth creation programs fail. Great ideas, but little to almost no practical ways to replicate it in everyday life.

This is where the *Inside-Out Wealth* approach truly shines. Using the tools of Neuro-Semantics, it is not only about your meanings, beliefs, and understandings of money, finances, value, creativity, business, creating wealth, etc. (your semantics), it is also about your actions, states, responses, and behavioral competencies (your neurological and physiological states)—your performances. It is about first winning the *inner game* and then about the *outer game* of finding a way to create value through your career and business.

What is Neuro-Semantics? The term literally refers to the embodiment (neuro-) of meanings (semantics). So as a model, it enables you to integrate your meanings and your performances. Using this model you will be invited to set critical *meanings* as mental frames about wealth, work, money, economics, business, etc. In this way you will set up your Inner Game so that you *think* like a millionaire. Doing that may require that you release various ideas or beliefs that don't support your creation of wealth. From there, you will begin to *embody* those meanings in your everyday activities so that you can *perform* the Outer Game of Wealth Creation and *act* like a millionaire.

Does the model work? Are you wondering—
> "Has it worked for the author? Has Dr. Hall become financially independent so that he has stopped working for money and become wealthy in all of the dimensions of wealth?"

The answer is yes. When I began this process I first set the goal of becoming financially independent. It took me six years to achieve that. Then, eight years from the day that I sat down and wrote my first Wealth Creation Plan, I accumulated my first million in equity in U.S. dollars. Do you know what's actually surprising about this? It just seemed to happen, it didn't require all the "work" that I had anticipated it would take. Like the people in one study that you'll discover, "It crept up on me."

While none of the secrets of wealth creation are rocket science, there is also not one of the secrets which is, in itself, "the" secret. There is no single panacea. The principles of wealth creating in today's world have been around in an explicit form for more than a century. This approach focuses on the *principles* as *the critical frames of mind* to empower you to think like a millionaire—yet that is just the beginning. Thinking like a millionaire is not enough. From there you have to *master yourself* so you can get yourself to actual *do* what you know, close the knowing-doing gap, and develop a practical plan for taking effective action.

Overview of Inside-Out Wealth
As an overview of what's in this book that will enable you to develop

Inside-Out Wealth, the book is divided into three parts.

Part I: The Dream. In this section I invite you to dream, to create your plan, to set your intentions, to identify the meanings and frames that will empower it, and to begin to get started. From this first section you will—
- Be inspired about what is possible by those who have created wealth and gain some significant understanding about wealth creation (chapter 1).
- Get an overview of the time frame and the seven stages of wealth creation (chapter 2).
- Set a high intention that will align your attentions to your highest values and purposes and develop an effective plan (chapter 3).
- Develop a clear understanding of what wealth is, its dimensions, and the kind of empowering beliefs that guide first-generation rich millionaires (chapter 4 and 5).

Part II: The Core. In this section, I will invite you to move from meaning into performance. Here you will —
- Get started by taking actions to handle your current job and money effectively and develop the required financial intelligence. This begins the process (chapter 6).
- Discover how *you* can use your gifts, skills, competencies, and passions to find a profitable source for identifying and creating value, combine into a synergy your talents and passions so that you find your singularity (chapter 7).
- Become a wealth creator in your identity so that your sense of self fully supports you in this process. Here you will also develop the inner wealth of who you are in your creativity, learning, joy, integrity, etc. Do this and then wealth will naturally flow from you and then to you (chapter 8).
- Identify those who you want to go with you in the wealth creation processes that you create. Wealth is never created alone; it is a collaboration between you and others. For that you'll need your support team of partners, colleagues, clients, suppliers, etc. Discover how to live with integrity as you create your business as you work with and through others (chapter 9).
- Figure out how to create a business out of your value proposition and build the systems in your business so that you can engage in the kind of entrepreneur-ing that will create multiple sources of income (chapter 10).

Part III: The Action States. The design of this section is to focus on the mind-body-emotional states that you will need to be able to translate your wealth creation plan into reality. Here you will—
- Identify and build enriching states for creating wealth from the inside-out. Then you will have ready access to the empowering states that will support and enhance your ability to handle the key factors involved in creating wealth. (Chapter 11)
- Identify the interference states that undermine your success, you will be able to escape "the matrix of frames" that creates that interference and so escape the "dragons" of impulsive spending, budgeting, saving, taking risks, investing etc. so that you don't stop yourself by various kinds of self-sabotage. (Chapter 12)
- Identify and create higher level states (meta-states) that will enable you to fully be a wealth creator. You will learn how to build such states of excellence as courage, resilience, persistence, self-efficacy, and efficiency. (Chapter 13)
- Build states of enjoyment so that the whole process is one of fun, excitement, and vitality. You will then have the passionate energy for being fully alive to your potentials. (Chapter 14)

While creating wealth involves motivation, the problem is not motivation. Motivation has its place, but you can be motivated and still uninformed and unskilled in the necessary skill set of practices to make it happen. That's why a *"Rah! Rah! I am a Millionaire!" Rally* will not do the trick; not in the long-term. You also have to know what "wealth" is, what creates it, and develop the practical financial skills to make it real.

So if this adventure is the one you've been waiting for, or if it is one that you are now ready for, then sit up, lower your tray table, get yourself ready to shift and change, expect lots of turbulence, and open wide your eyes to the possibilities for inside-out wealth!

Your Wealth Coach
Each chapter ends with an invitation for you. If you will take me on as your Wealth Coach, then I will facilitate the processes from that chapter for you to experience *Your Wealth Creation Adventure.* Then you will be empowered to take your next steps in creating wealth and unleashing your Wealth Creator self. To prepare for this, get a notebook and on it inscribe the words— *Wealth Creation Adventure Journal.*

Notes:
1. Financial independence is not a description of how much money you have, it's a description of the fact that you don't *have to* go to work to live. You are *independent* of depending on working for your basic life-style. Your money now works for you giving you the lifestyle you want and the freedom to explore, contribute, and be according to your personal values and visions.

PART I

THE DREAM OF

WEALTH CREATION

**May you become a Dreamer in the Day
and translate your dream
into your everyday actions!**

Chapter 1

CAN WEALTH

BE CREATED?

- Is it possible for you to just decide, "I'm going to become a wealth creator and create wealth for myself and others!" and to make it so?
- If you did make a decision like that, what would you then do? How would you then go about creating wealth?

With so many people who live in constant financial stress and with the media suggesting that we believe that we live in a world of scarcity governed by the economic theory that "the pie is only so large," and so the more people helping themselves means that there's less for everybody else. So how *can* we *create* wealth? Is that really possible?

If wealth can be created, why don't more people actually do that? What stops people from becoming financially independent? *How* can you become smarter about handling your finances and creating of wealth so you stop working for money and get money to work for you?

If the problem is not the lack of opportunity, then what explains the lack of financial freedom and financial independence? Why do so many people have so much stress over finances and struggle to make ends meet? Could it be that you are not internally and personally organized in your mind-and-emotions for wealth creation? Could it simply be that you do not have the proper frames of mind for wealth?

The fact is that even smart people make big mistakes about money. They either sell their souls for it, let money define who they are and "the good life," or they have a mistaken mental map, a mental map that doesn't guide them as they navigate work, career, speaking, etc. Without having an accurate and workable map for creating wealth, you will join the ranks of the talented, intelligent, and gifted *poor* people of the world.

My Personal Story
I know this works because of my own personal story. I was in my late thirties when I finally realized that money was important afterall. At the time, realizing that was a revelation! It was a revelation because I had spent 17 years of my adult life (21 to 38) in professions that were highly *people centered*. My focus, interests, and passions were not about money, financial success, or "success" in terms of status, cars, homes, clothes, etc. As a minister, a psychotherapist, and then as a psychologist, I had a different focus—my focus was to understand and help people make changes to improve the quality of their lives.

In fact, if you had asked about what I thought about money during those years, I would have answered from a blur of consciousness and with convoluted statements:
> "Yeah, it's important—for paying bills and taking care of business; but it is also a big problem, most people are too greedy and overly focused on money. Life is about so much more."

Depending on when during the month you would have asked me, I would have also complained about being in a low-paying profession, of living paycheck to paycheck, or of things costing too much. If you had asked me how money works, how wealth is created, how economies work, how to think like an entrepreneur, successful components of business, how to save and invest, or other such questions, I would have effectively demonstrated my ignorance. I didn't know. And worse, I really didn't care about knowing! I had bigger fish to fry. I had not studied anything that would have provided me answers. I didn't even know how to buy a house, how to work with banks to get a mortgage. I was ignorant about all of that and worse, I was also ignorant of the depth of my ignorance! I was in a state of bliss—delightful, ego-satisfying, and stupifying. Ah, those were the days!

The one saving grace was that I knew how to save what little I had. In fact, I had been saving for years. That was one thing I had learned how to do. I learned it first through the example that my dad gave me. He had lived through the Great Depression of the 1930s and then he spent his life in low-paying profession as a mathematics teacher at the high school. I also learned the same as I similarly chose to enter low-pay professions in my twenties and thirties and so I had to learn how to get by on little. Later when I married, I had $9,000 saved and so a few years later, my wife and I were able to buy our first house for $34,000 in 1986 having saved for years to be able to make a down payment of eleven thousand. The next year she left, so I was faced with a divorce and legal fees in fighting for custody of our daughter. When all the dust settled, I was 38, a single dad raising a 3-year old with no child support from my ex-wife, and had a grand total of $500 to my name. Ah, the fruits of my ignorance!

That's when I had my first eureka moment and arrived at the radical conclusion: "Hey, money is important afterall!" I also made a decision:
> "Never again would I put myself or find myself in a position where I have to start all over again. Never again will I be reduced to zero. I will learn how to become financially stable."

Yes, my first wealth creation decision was *an away-from decision* —away from what I didn't want. All I want then was some financial *stability*. Several years later I would make another formative decision, a *toward decision* of becoming financially independent so that I could choose how I wanted to live. But the *away-from decision* was enough to get started. In the coming chapters I'll tell about the episodes that followed: investing in my self-development, buying my first investment property, using frugality in the early stages, and so on.

Modeling Wealth
I began modeling the structure, stages, and processes of creating wealth in the mid-1990s by interviewing several wealthy individuals who were very successful in their respected areas. I interviewed a contractor builder worth $19 million, a movie producer and advertizer who had accumulated $4 million by the age of 30, and the owner of a seat belt company who was worth $12 million. I began with my personal friend, Tom Beam of Oklahoma City, who had the seat belt company, and then

some acquaintances with whom I met through various business arrangements. There were several others as well.

Seven interviews later, I was significantly disappointed. That's when I realized my first mistake. I had been interviewing people successful in finances without setting up any criteria for what counted as "success." What I discovered was that while a person could be successful in accumulating money, that did not mean success in keeping it or attaining it in an ecological way. I discovered that some of the people I interviewed had strategies for generating money that I would never use. The way they did it and the costs they paid for doing it, was not something I wanted.

For example, several made their fortune at the cost of their relationships. At 76 years of age, the contractor's grown children would not even talk to him! One did so at the cost of his health, working 14 to 16 hour days and under tremendous stress. Another one made his wealth by engaging in ethically questionable practices and always looking over his shoulder worried about getting caught.

The first interviews caught me by surprise and taught me to set some criteria. I wanted to learn the secrets of first-generation rich who created it ethically by contributing value in a healthful way. I wanted to study the lives of those who built businesses around their contribution so that it would have a life of its own and be making money even when the person wasn't there.

Soon thereafter my frustration paid dividends. It happened when I did something really radical—I made a trip to the my local library! I went there on an adventure—to see if anyone had ever research this area, and if so, what they found. I didn't even know if there would be a field of literature on this subject. Was I surprised!

As I found the section in the library for the books on finance and wealth creation, I suddenly discovered that there was a whole library of studies, longitudinal studies, studies of hundreds if not thousands of people.

NLP — A Communication Model based on two world-class communicators using the distinctions of Transformational Grammar to create a model of how language works in human neurology to create our experiences (states) of reality.

I discovered that there were rows of books that had been exploring and examining first-generation rich millionaires. And best of all—all this information was there—unsorted, unclassified, and in the raw. As such. it was not all that useful—the presentation mostly framed in very vague generalizations—as "principles" or "laws" of wealth creation. Yet the information was just sitting there on the shelves ready to be modeled using the modeling tools of NLP and Neuro-Semantics. And that's precisely what I did.

When I say that the information was there "in the raw," I mean that the books described who made a fortune, and when and where they became wealthy. They described what the person did and even how they did it. Lots of raw data, but with very little structural form to make it useful. And that's what made it ineffective and unuseable.

Imagine a reporter describing Tiger Woods playing golf. The data is all there and it's a great story—quite inspiring. And in a general way we would know what to do to play like Tiger—believe in yourself, get a mentor, and practice hitting golf balls for years, in fact, practice for decades! But really, how helpful is that? We might even get a few peeks into his mind— some of his ideas, beliefs, and strategies. That would help, but again, how helpful would that be if our goal is to become a world-class golfer like him?

> **Neuro-Semantics (NS):** A model of human meaning, how we create meaning within our brain and neurology, and then perform that meaning (or at least attempt to) in our body, emotions, and behaviors.
>
> **Meta-States:** A model of the unique form of human consciousness— self-reflexive consciousness, how the mind reflects on itself to create layers of meanings as *frames* of mind.

The data has to be *modeled* and that's where *the modeling tools* of Neuro-Semantics comes in. Now modeling requires numerous things; breaking down the skills and competencies into sub-strategies, identifying the stages and steps in learning how to practice the strategies, and how to put them together as a whole, and then even remodeling the strategies to customize it to a new person and context.

As I read fifty books on the subject, I eventually found a few key researchers that I began to primarily rely upon in building the *Inside-Out Wealth* program. The key researchers that I focused on include Scrully Blotnick, Thomas Stanley and William Danko, Robert Kiyosaki, Robert Allen, and Suze Orman. There were others, but these were the key thinkers. From them I modeled out a strategy for wealth creation. The next step was to try on the strategy and the sub-strategies myself to see if they worked and how well they worked. Could I make them work? Once I was convinced because it was working for me, I began training the process. That began in 1999. In that year I went to New York City, London, and several other places. Since then, *Inside-Out Wealth* has been presented in the US, England, France, Moscow Russia (several times), Australia, South Africa, and many other places.

Modeling
As mentioned, the Inside-Out Wealth process was modeled from both live examples and the literature of wealth researchers— their longitudinal studies of people who created wealth. *NLP modeling* originated from the field of Cognitive-Behavioral psychology. It began with the work of George Miller and his associates as revealed in *The Plan and Structure of Behavior* (1960). In that work, they presented the TOTE model to explain how our minds and bodies respond to things and build strategies for either coping or mastering a competency.

TOTE—Test-Operate-Test-Exit—enabled the first researchers to begin identifying what goes on *inside* a person's mind to create the right state for doing something. We **T**est an action to see if it reaches an outcome. If not, we **O**perate to change our action or our objective.

> **Modeling:** The process of identifying the component elements of an experience and putting them into a form that can be used to replicate the skills, expertise, or excellence.

We then **T**est again to see what happened, and if it succeeded, we **E**xit the process. TOTE applies to the smallest of actions and to some larger behaviors.

You can use this model to describe the behavior of such things like "tuning a radio." Using a criteria of what's desired (the targeted outcome), you *test* what you see or hear as when you tune a radio into a station. If the radio is not on the station, you turn the knob this way or that until it sounds like it is on the station and when you no longer hear any static. That's the *testing* and the *operating* actions. The next *test* is seeing if what you did worked and how well did it work. If it does not, then more *operating* (adjusting the knob). If it does, then *exiting* the process.

Richard Bandler and John Grinder, the co-founders of NLP, took this TOTE model and added the representation systems to it. This created the Strategies Model for modeling. Robert Dilts wrote the foundational NLP book on this, *NLP: The Study of the Structure of Subjective Experience* (1980), and later another book on *NLP Modeling*.

The Strategies Model enables us to identify the step-by-step process for micro-behaviors like spelling, getting motivated to get out of bed, making a decision, etc. Micro-behaviors are those behaviors that occur within a short period of time (typically in a few minutes).

When expert spellers were modeled, it was discovered that when they heard a word spoken (external stimuli), they would *represent* that word by making an *internal picture* of it (see it on the screen of their mind) and *test* it against a previously stored picture of the word. If the representation fit the test, there would be no *operation* on it. If it did not fit, they would *operate* by changing the image in their mind. They would then *test* the new *visual image of the word* that they have heard and if it *felt* right (kinesthetic sensation of "right" rather than "wrong"), then they would *exit* this program. If it did not feel right or if it felt wrong, they would loop back to *operating* again and do so until it felt right so they could *exit*.

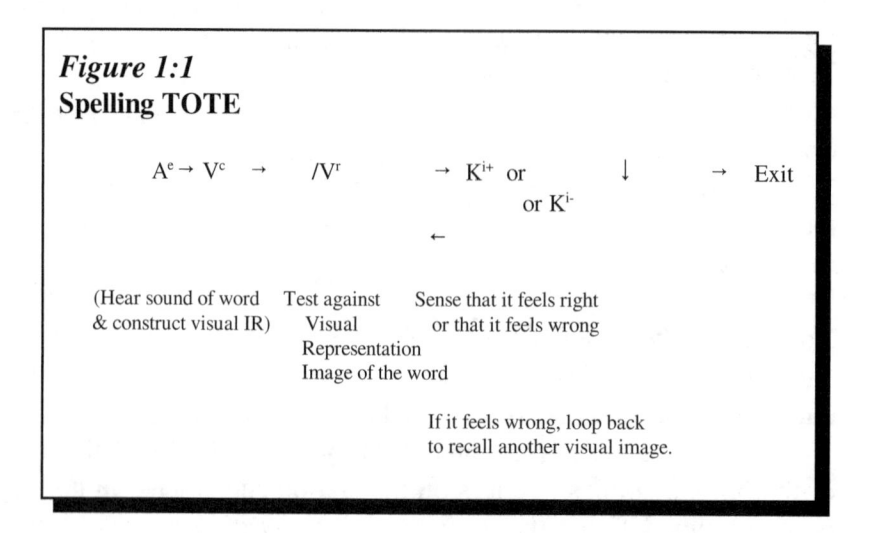

Figure 1:1
Spelling TOTE

$A^e \rightarrow V^c \rightarrow /V^r \rightarrow K^{i+}$ or $\downarrow \rightarrow$ Exit
or K^{i-}

$\leftarrow$

(Hear sound of word   Test against   Sense that it feels right
& construct visual IR)   Visual   or that it feels wrong
                          Representation
                          Image of the word

                                         If it feels wrong, loop back
                                         to recall another visual image.

NLP modeling. And it works great for micro-behaviors. But what about more complex behaviors—behaviors that occur over a longer-period of time, days, weeks, months, and even years? How do we model something like that? And what about activities like wealth creation that involves many, many behaviors over much longer periods of time? For this we need not only the step-by-step process, we also need the vertical levels that layer our mind with the required mental contexts.

This is where the Meta-States Model comes in. I discovered and formulated that model in 1994 while modeling Resilience. I discovered that resilience is not just a step-by-step process, but involves several stages and involves higher level states.[1]

Meta-State modeling enables you to move up vertically to the higher self-reflexive thinking of a person's mind. This modeling goes upward (vertically) as well as outward (horizontally). And as such it enables you to model an *attitude* as well as a skill or set of behaviors. I'll explain more about this as we progress in the following chapters and in the three chapters on the *states* of wealth creation (chapters 11-13), we will use the Meta-States Model to create and install great wealth creation attitudes that you can carry with you for the rest of your life.

Blotnick's *Getting Rich Your Own Way* (1980)
Beginning in 1960 Scrully Blotnick, Ph.D. identified and then followed 1,500 people who wanted to get rich. Over the years he lost one-third of the participants in the project. Yet from the remaining 1,057 people, 83 became millionaires. He and his associates then interviewed more than 200 multi-millionaires to discover the secrets of becoming wealthy.
> "We are not going to make matters worse by telling you we've found a secret formula that will make you rich overnight. There is no such thing, though we know plenty of people who've gone broke looking for it. What we are about to describe might be labeled a 'get rich slow' technique. But it works. And nothing else does." (p. 15)

As it turned out, this "get rich slow" technique was a common theme among all the researchers. For Blotnick, his longitudinal research led him to identify two key stages in wealth creation which he named as the absorbed and the investment stages.

Stage I: The Profoundly Absorbed Stage.
>In the first stage the people invested primarily in themselves, their learning and skills as they found an absorbing interest or skill, and gave themselves to it. Those who ultimately became rich were profoundly absorbed by a particular activity. Thanks to the fact that they were so caught up in it, they persisted in it and so eventually excelled at it. Time and energy is invested in oneself, in your education, development, skills, and growth.

Stage II: The Investment Stage.
>In the second stage those who became wealthy began to invest the money that they had been making. They became investors because the activity they excelled at produced more income than they could invest in themselves. Now time and energy was devoted to investing money into stocks, bonds, CDs, real estate, etc.

Stage one is the key to the creation of wealth. In this work, I am calling it *inside-out wealth* because it is the personal wealth of a passion and a set of competencies that allow you to become engaged in something—that with enough time, effort, persistence, learning, resilience, etc.— will enable you to create a fortune.

>"What characterized developing millionaires is that they unintentionally proceeded from Stage One to Stage Two. What characterized people who failed was that they intentionally tried— repeatedly—to go from Stage Two to Stage One. Few ever made it out of Stage Two. Are you surprised that they were—and still are so frustrated, anxious, and annoyed?" (p. 51)

>"The vast majority of people make things much worse for themselves by trying to go from Stage 2 to Stage 1, from first finding financial independence to subsequently locating an absorbing interest. . . . They want Stage 1 *and* Stage 2 simultaneously! But no one can hand you Stage 1 Satisfaction. You have to find that yourself. Profound involvement in an area always springs from sources deep within a person (pp. 90-91)

And when asked about the value and meaningfulness of the two stages, Stage One always won out.

>"Which of the two stages meant more to the people who became millionaires? None had to even think about the answer. It was Stage One." (p. 50)

The state of being fully engaged in doing something that you care about, that you believe in, that you are willing to learn, persist in, and become competent in is the key to creating a foundation for wealth creation. Blotnick discovered that it was the power of engagement that seemed to be one of the most important features. Here are some of his reflections about this:

"A child's desire to be hypnotically engrossed doesn't end with childhood. Being absorbed is deeper and more important than like and dislike, love and hate. It is the only magic our everyday lives have left. ... Those who were better at becoming absorbed by their work looked forward to being caught up in it and also found it inherently rewarding (p. 202, 212)

If you want a secret of wealth creation, here is one: *absorption.* Let something absorb your interests, your passions, your skills, your direction in life and let that absorption become your focus state wherein you create value for others. Do that and you are well on your way to inside-out wealth. In Neuro-Semantics we call this flow state of intense focus and engagement a "genius" state.[2]

Blotnick identified this psychological state of absorption as the dynamic that turned every day work into a source of wealth creation:

"A missing ingredient, a key one which operates so quietly it had previously been overlooked, had to be present if someone was ever to become rich: *they had to find their work absorbing. Involving. Enthralling.*" (p. 6)

The personal power that this state of absorption facilitates is the power of enjoyment. Joyful absorption enables you to do whatever it is that you do joyfully and when you do that, you are not "working." You are expending energy, sometimes tremendous energy, like a child playing at something, and why is that important? This eliminates most of the stress that typically characterizes work. It is no longer drudgery.

"As it turns out, your work is more likely to make you wealthy than any bet or investment that you ever make. ... *The crucial role played by work you enjoy* is only one of the startling conclusions which emerged. There were others." (p. 5).

This will become increasingly clear in the coming chapters and the focus of Part II on the core of wealth creation. Surprisingly, almost all of those who eventually became millionaires hardly noticed it. Blotnick's words were succinct: "Basically, it crept up on them." (p. 37).

Were there any specific personality traits or qualities in those who became rich? Blotnick reduced the qualities to the following five:

> 1) *Persistent* in a field or activity that they stick with through good times and bad as they became passionate in that which they became absorbed in.
> 2) *Patient* in being willing to wait forever, if necessary, for the rewards of one's labors.
> 3) *Accepted* the pettier and trivial aspects of the job, didn't reject as "beneath" them.
> 4) *Collaborative* with others, and less competitive attitude toward people with whom they worked.
> 5) *Only minimally focused on investment activities.* Only consumed a minimum of time and attention. (pp. 6-7)

Absorption also means something else. It means that you no longer have a job, you have a mission. Being absorbed means experiencing a "flow" state of such intense concentration that time goes away, the world goes away, everything disappears except the subject of your engagement. This again describes the genius state and explains why I have devoted Part III to developing this state, along with many other critical states for wealth creation.

Another important discovery arose from this research, namely, that wealth is created by valuing and appreciating the ordinary values of life rather than over-valuing status and wealth symbols.

> "*Why* do so many people overlook economic opportunities? One reason has to do with social status?" (p. 193)

Blotnick noted that a great many people typically *discount* such blue-collar businesses like owning a junkyard, pawn shop, car wash business, fast food franchise, and so on.

> "The intense need for social status blinds people to many significant economic opportunities. Snobs do not make great entrepreneurs. (p. 194)

I began with Blotnick's research and his data. It offered me a great start and enabled me to do what he did not, namely, track specific beliefs, strategies, and meta-states of those who became wealthy.[3] I began with the key behaviors he identified and supplemented with those he missed. I began with the key mis-beliefs and mis-understandings he identified and added more that I and others found.

Stanley and Danko's Millionaire Research

Researchers Thomas Stanley and William Danko began their research with an exploration regarding *where to find* the self-made first-generation rich millionaires. Surely they live in the upscale subdivisions outside the urban city areas, right? Wrong! In fact, that idea turned out to be completely wrong. Instead they live next door. They live in 25-year old homes. And that led to the title of their first book—*The Millionaire Next Door* (1996, 2001).

> "Snobs do not make great entrepreneurs."
> Blotnick

This was surprising and it led to many other surprising conclusions about the wealthy. Stanley and Danko began their exploration with many questions about these first-generation rich millionaires—their saving habits, their enjoyment of their work, their lifestyle habits, their habitual ways of thinking, and much more. A few years later Stanley published a follow-up work, *The Millionaire Mind* (2000).

In the first book they distinguished two types of people in terms of accumulating wealth—PAW and UAW and the difference in their values and style of living.

> "The Prodigious Accumulators of Wealth (PAW) love working, while a large proportion of Under Accumulators of Wealth (UAW) work because they need to support their conspicuous consumption habit. Money should never change one's values ... Making money is only a report card. It's a way to tell how you're doing." (*The Millionaire Next Door,* p. 110)

Through their extensive research about the life-style of the first-generation rich millionaires, they discovered numerous things such as the importance of character:

> "After 20 years of studying millionaires, we have concluded that *the character* of the business owner is more important in predicting his level of wealth than the classification of his business." (p. 228)

These studies provide a tremendous amount of data about the mindsets, attitudes, and lifestyle of those who became wealthy. So I will often refer to these research studies in the coming chapters.[4]

Robert Kiyosaki's Research

Robert Kiyosaki packaged his exploration into this field—into money, income, saving, investing, creating wealth, etc.—in terms of his personal experience with his two "dads." In his best selling book, *Rich Day, Poor Day* he frames two ways of thinking about and handling money. *Poor dad* was his actual dad, *rich dad* was the father of his best friend. The first dad approached wealth as an employee and so had eyes for security, for avoidance of risk, and for how to become wealthy through income. The second dad approached wealth as an entrepreneur and so the world of business and money through the eyes of opportunities, adding value, and increasing his entrepreneurial competencies. The first dad became poor, the second dad became wealthy.

Figure 1:2

Left Side	*Right Side*
S	**I**
Self-Employee	**Investor**
We own a job	Capitalize on other
Independent	Businesses
Make $ from work	
Creative	
Active	
E	**B**
Employee	**Business**
We have a job	Activity occurs
Dependent on boss	beyond individual.
$ from job	System has life of its own.
Receive	Automated
Passive	Systematized

While his *poor dad* was well-educated and intelligent (e.g., he had a Ph.D. in education), he worked for someone else, believed in security more than informed risk-taking, feared the idea of going out on his own, and so he *worked for money*. By contrast, his best friend's dad was not well-educated (in terms of university degrees), but he was highly intelligent in terms of creating wealth and entrepreneur-ing. He believed that the riskiest thing in the world was to work for someone else, he believed that unlimited money could be made if one knew how to add value and seize opportunities. In his case, *money worked for him.*

To understand how money is made, Robert Kiyosaki designed a model of Cash Flow Quadrants and divided it between left side and right side (see *Cash Flow Quadrants*). On the left side, the earning process is based on the formula of "time for money." You get paid when you work, when you contribute, and when you are at the business. When you move to the right side of the quadrants, money works for you. Your business or your investments is now able to make money for you even when you are not there.

Because I'll refer to the cashflow quadrants in the coming chapters, I've included Figure 1:2 —the quadrants by which you can identify the source of your income.

Robert Allen's Wealth Through Real Estate

Robert Allen caught my attention for two reasons, first because he had worked for awhile with Richard Bander, co-founder of NLP, and second, because his area of expertise was in real estate. So in *Wealth Creation* and in *No Money Down in the 80s (in the 90s, etc.)* he developed a four-stage process for creating wealth. The basic format involves the meta-strategy of thinking long-term:
      1) Getting started
      2) Creating capital
      3) Investing capital
      4) Protecting capital

A great deal of Robert Allen's work focuses on both the false assumptions and beliefs that undermine wealth that must be recognized and dealt with before taking on the useful ideas that lead to success in creating wealth.
      "Wealth is not money. Money is just the appearance of wealth. The form, but not the substance. Wealth is thoughts, not things. ... Wealth

is a state of mind—an attitude." (1983, p. 18)

"The last thing that people want to hear is the plain simple fact that the rich think differently than the poor. They are programmed differently. They have different expectations with respect to money. They have a wealthy mindset. It is as if there were a filter between you and your world— the filter of your mind." (p. 21)

Modeling Wealth Creators

So, what can we learn from all of these efforts in modeling wealth creators?

- What does the research on the first-generation rich self-made millionaires show?
- What secrets have come to light through the study of people who have been successful in creating wealth, who have not ruined their health or relationships in doing so, and who have done so ethically and in ways that make their lives richer in every way?
- Is there a structure to the process of creating wealth and sustaining that wealth?

The answer to the last question is easy: "Yes, there is a structure, a strategy, and it can be learned and replicated." And the answer to the first two questions is more involved and will take up the rest of this book.

Here is the overall strategy of Inside-Out Wealth the secret of the wealth creation approach that follows:

Find a passion that you can invest yourself into fully with fascination, engagement, and joy. Then invest in your mind and self-development so that you develop your skills into masterful competencies so that you can add value in a domain or niche that has the potential for creating lots of money.

Invest in your own financial and wealth education so that you handle your money wisely as you save, budget, and invest. As you explore and transform your innate talents into skilled competencies, bring persistence and resilience to your vision and plan so that you can stay with it as it mature into financial independence and wealth.

With your singularity of potential, passion, and profit, *develop your valued competencies into an expertise that satisfies your market.* As you develop your business sense, get the right people on the bus with you and set up the systems so that the business develops a life of its own. *Now persist for a decade.* Handle all the ups-and-downs with vitality and resilience and keep learning from feedback in a way that keeps your vision and passion alive. Then before you know it, wealth will creep up on you!

This is the "get rich slowly" process that Blotnick mentioned, and it works. It is also based on the *inside out wealth* principle. First you focus on yourself (your *being* wealth) so that *you* in yourself become abundantly wealth. You have value that you contribute and that people will pay for. That self-investment of competence, expertise, and mastery in what you know and can do for others then leads to your *doing* wealth— your valued skill, competency, and mastery that solves one or more problems. Your *doing* wealth means that you can meet the needs of customers in a given niche or domain. It means you can supply a valued desire of people. Then with your *being* and *doing* wealth inside you— you can translate that by entering or inventing a business. This leads to your *having* wealth—the money, equity, business ownership, and all of the stuff that money can buy.

> **Be:** Your inner wealth of mind, emotion, and person. The wealth of who you are.
>
> **Do:** The wealth of what you can do and achieve through your powers of mind, emotion, speech, and behavior. The contribution you make as you add value to others.
>
> **Have:** The wealth of the stuff that you obtain, money, houses, cars, clothes, and all of the toys that make life easier and more enjoyable. The stuff that you have to give and contribute, and to leave as a legacy of the difference you can make in the world.

Inside-out wealth is a wealth creation approach that calls upon you to unleash your financial genius, your creativity, your business acumen, and your ability to find and release your unique gifts. It is about actualizing your highest and best.

Inside-out wealth includes your *experiential* wealth—the richness of the experiences that you value: the contribution you make, the problems you solve, the difference you make, the discoveries you make, the learnings, the wisdom, the care, the love, and the value that you add. And in the end, you have *legacy* wealth—the wealth that you leave as you make your mark on the world.

Back to the Biggest Wealth Creation Myth
If there is any one thing that can get in your way and sabotage your efforts—it is the seduction of the "Get Rich Quick" mentality. This must be recognized for what it is and firmly, even stubbornly, refused. I hope it is obvious by now that the kind of multi-dimensional wealth that inside-out wealth refers to cannot be created, developed, or enjoyed with the get-rich-quick mentality. That way of thinking and the feelings that it generates (impatience, stress, pressure, greed, fear, etc.) leads to playing the wrong game. As a strategy, it does not work.

The get-rich-quick mentality is the same mentality that also defeats and undermines lottery winners. The great majority of people (60 to 90 percent) who experience a win-fall through the lottery are not able to keep the money. Not only that, they are not prepared for the money and so don't know how to handle it. Within three years, most have lost it all. But worst, in those years, they have been personally devastated by their own internal unpreparedness to handle the responsibilities that money brings them. They have lost friends and loved-ones, they have given up their jobs and don't know what to do with their lives.

It is *long-term strategic thinking* that creates solid and lasting wealth. That's why a key secret for inside-out wealth is to think about the process in terms of building wealth over a decade. When you do that, then you will recognize the natural stages and be able to handle those stages of wealth creation. Then you will be able to keep asking the strategic questions of yourself:
> Where am I in my ten-year wealth creation process? What skills and states do I need to fully develop for this stage? What will be those that will take me to the next level? What counts that I can enjoy and celebrate at this stage?

In the *inside-out wealth* approach, another insightful secret is this: *money is just a scorecard*. Money is not wealth, it is only a sign and indicator of wealth. This attitude, rather than devaluing money, puts money into its proper place. You can now use money as a measurement and as a tool, without making wealth creation solely about money. Wealth is about so much more than money. It is about *living* from an abundant mind and emotion. It is about *being* wealthy on your inside so that there's no sense of poverty in yourself or what you can do or what you can offer or what you can enjoy.

In this I think you also recognize another secret, namely that *wealth creation is strategic.* It is highly strategic. That's why typically it does not just happen to good people, intelligent people, or well-intentioned people. Sure there are the winfalls that sometimes occur and sure, there are situations when someone happens upon a fortune. But for the great majority of people, that's not how it happens.

Inside-out wealth is an approach that enables you to become an *intentional* wealth creator. And this approach is based upon finding and using your unique singularity. This *singularity* of wealth creation that Jim Collins and William Porras discovered in *Good to Great* about companies is the same for individuals. It is the interface of three things: Passion, Potential, and Profit. It is strategic about developing your value and contribution first and how to interface with a market and need.

Finally, the inside-out wealth approach adds something unique to wealth creation that the key thinkers and researchers know, but often do not make explicit enough. Namely, *wealth and wealth creation are psychological phenomena.* From beginning to end, *creating wealth entails your personal psychology* (thoughts and emotions) about money, economics, skills and competencies, supply and demand, business, responsibility, frames of mind, resourceful states, working with and through others, psychology of selling, positioning, and much more. Not only that, but "wealth" itself is as much a psychological state as it is a financial state. That's why there are rich people (according to their bank accounts) who are poor inside—paranoid, stingy, miserly, selfish, ego-centric, etc. And who wants those states?

The *inside-out wealth* approach here is psychologically healthy and whole. It enables you to *be* wealthy in mind, emotions, speech, behavior, relationships, time, attitude, etc. Inside-out wealth is truly an *inside*

> Not only that, but "wealth" itself is as much a psychological state as it is a financial state.

phenomena first. It is learning to *be* wealthy within—that enables you to find, create, and celebrate the creation of value. It enables you to create a set of wealthy states of commitment, investment, patience, joy, networking, supporting, listening, seeing with your mind's eye of opportunities to add value. It enables you to be wealthy in *doing* as you actually translate what you know into what you do and so close the knowing-doing gap. And that makes you rich in being able to make things happen.

Your Adventure in Creating Wealth
Are you ready for a conversation with your wealth coach? If so, then I want to invite you to begin today creating your wealth creation plan and adventure. To do that, review the highlights of this chapter and identify the key ideas or principles that you want for your experience of wealth creation. Make a list. Chapter 15 of this book is designed to give you a plan to begin creating your personalized *Inside-Out Wealth Creation Plan*.

From your lists identify the top three ideas—the three ideas that would make a transformational difference in your life. Transfer these three ideas to a 3-by-5 card or piece of paper that you can carry with you everywhere you go for the next week. Use the card to constantly (once an hour) remind yourself of these guiding ideas.

End of Chapter Notes
1. See *Meta-States* (2008) for the resilience strategy. There is also a training manual with the title, Resilience. Also on modeling is the book: *NLP Going Meta* (2008).

2: A "genius" state is a state of full engagement so that you develop a single-minded focus. See *Secrets of Personal Mastery* and *the APG training manual or workshop.*

3. See Blotnick's other books such as *Winning: The Psychology of Successful Investing. Ambitious Men* (1987).

4. Other books by Thomas include *The Millionaire Mind* (2000), *The Millionaire Women Next Door* (2004).

5. Robert Kiyosaki, *Rich Dad; Poor Dad.* (1992). *Cash Flow Quadrants* (1998).

6. Robert Allen. *Getting Rich in the 90s.*

Chapter 2

HOW LONG WILL IT TAKE?

"Thinking to get at once all the gold the goose could give,
he killed it, and opened it only to find— nothing."
Aesop

"Being rich isn't a passive state. Ultimately, time is more valuable than money, because if you run out of money, you can start over agin. But when you run out of time, there's no starting over. . . . Billionaires never wish away the minutes; life's just too good to wish it away. Be present in time, fully engaged."
Donald Trump

"You won't achieve your financial goals
if you don't behave like a long-term investor."
Jonathan Clements (1998, p. 152)

Okay, so if the *inside-out wealth* approach is not a get-rich-quick scheme, how long will it take? What are we actually talking about here in terms of time? And why? Why can't it be quick? Why does the creation of wealth take so much time? How quickly can you become wealthy? How patient or impatient are you to become a wealth creator? How much time will you give yourself to become financially independent? What plans have you developed for your wealth creating?

The *Why* of the Time Length
I'll answer the *why question* first. It takes a long time because there are numerous stages in the process—stages that involve the development of

your core competencies. Unless someone just comes up and hands you a check for a million dollars, then *you* have to *create* something that people want and for which they will invest their money. And if you have to *create something of value,* then you have to develop the knowledge and skills to create that something. What will it be? And that means developing the required competencies which will have the quality that will make your contribution valuable. And once you have done all of that, then you have to create or find a business context so that you can use your expertise, make it known, sell it, distribute it, collect the money, etc. And all of that development requires time.

> **The Stage Principle:**
> *Wealth is best built in stages; it is not built in a moment or overnight.*

Talents turned into skills, skills turned into competencies, turned into expertise—all require time. There is no such thing as "instant competence" or "instant expertise." And to figure out which of your competencies to devote yourself to—with sufficient passion and persistence— that also requires time. It takes experimenting, testing, trying different things. Then once you know your passion and potential expertise, you also have to find "an economic engine" —a practical means for making money. And again, that takes time. And all of this explains *why* the get-rich-quick mentality and approach not only does not work, but actually undermines the wealth creation process. If it was that quick and that easy, everybody would be a millionaire. But obviously, everyone is not.

The Stage Factor
Given that it takes all of that and more, there are numerous stages in the process. For purposes of a clarifying focus, I have separated out *seven stages* inherent in the *inside-out wealth* approach. Over the time frame of these seven stages, you will identify what and how you will create wealth and then focus on the wealth creation engagement itself.

Now given that there are *stages* in the wealth creation process, the key to effectively navigating these stages requires understanding each stage and giving each stage empowering meanings. Ultimately, it is the meanings and intentions that you construct about each stage that governs how you unleash your wealth creation potentials at any given stage. Inadequate and wrong meanings will cause you to become stuck at any given stage where adequate meanings will empower you to succeed. At each stage you will need to awaken or create rich and robust meanings. Doing that will then enable you to respond effectively in your wealth performances.

`Figure 2:1

Actualizing your highest and best wealth creation throughout the stages requires two things. It requires your highest *meanings* and your best *performances*. That's because actualizing your highest and best (self-actualization) is a function of these two factors. So to unleash your wealth creation potentials, it has to be meaningful to you (significance, valuable, your vision and mission) and you have to be able to perform it in actions (your skills, competence, expertise, and mastery).[1]

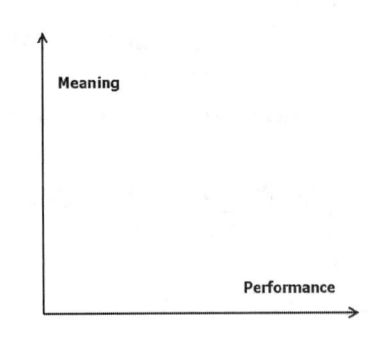

How long will it take? To a great extent it depends on what stage you are in at this moment as well as how long you take to progress to the next stage. It depends on the number of changes you will have to make, your skill and speed at changing, and it also depends on the external market and the people you have to work with and through. So given all that, are you ready for the seven stages?

    1) Preparation
    2) Singularity
    3) Collaboration
    4) Business Launch
    5) Business Development Strategy
    6) Investment
    7) Exit

Now to facilitate and model the wealth creation process, I will use the Matrix Model.[2] This modeling tool from Neuro-Semantics enables us to sort out three process matrices by which you create your sense of reality (meaning, intention, and state) and five content matrices that contain the information and stories that you carry with you and use as filters for your experiences (self, power, others, time, world).

The term "matrix" here refers to how you transform your referent events and experiences into your internal frames of reference— your inner frames of mind. And within your frames of mind are incorporated the meanings that you have inherited, absorbed, and invented—your interpretations of things and your interpretative style. Your internal matrix of frames then determine, govern, and filter your experiences.

> **The Seven Stages of Wealth Creation**
> 1) Preparation
> 2) Singularity
> 3) Collaboration
> 4) Business Launch
> 5) Business Development Strategy
> 6) Investment
> 7) Exit

You can call the meaning frames that make up your Matrix your "beliefs, understandings, or ideas." Your matrix is the inner world that you live in and that you most often and commonly (like the rest of us) confuse with reality. And that's important.

Why? How? It's important because all of your "problems" are functions of your frames, not reality. People who have problems with "money," "wealth," "budgeting," "saving," etc. do not have problems with certain external events or activities. What they actually have trouble with is *their ideas and therefore feelings about* those things, events, and activities. It is *how they interpret and therefore experience* those events that is a problem. So the problem is always the frame, and never the person. And knowing that means that the place for change, for transformation, for intervention is not in the

> **The Matrix Model**
> *Process matrices:*
>   Meaning
>   Intention
>   State
> *Content matrices:*
>   Self
>   Power
>   Others
>   Time
>   World

things, activities, or experiences of the world— but in your *interpretations* of it. This will become increasingly clear as we progress through the chapters.[3]

We use the Matrix Model in Neuro-Semantics as a systems model to help sort out the complexity of an experience and to follow *the information—energy circuits.* This refers to how you take in information and then through your processing of that information turn it into signals and commands to your neurology thereby incorporating and embodying that information so that it becomes part and parcel of your muscle memory. In this, *information* literally *in-forms* you—it *forms* you *on the inside,* making you who you are, how you feel, and how you function. What information currently *informs* you? Does that information enhance your life? Therefore your emotions and actions are functions of your matrix of frames and therefore symptoms rather than causes. That is, how you feel and what you do are governed and directed by your frames.[4]

Wealth Creation Time-Line

Matrices

Intention / Meaning

Powers Self   Others   World

    Saving $
    Work   Profit
                 Passion
   States   Potential

I	II	III	IV	V	VI	VII
Preparation	Singularity	Collaboration	Business Launch	Development Strategy	Investment	Exit

Robert Kiyosaki:

  Employee   *Self-Employed*   *Business Owner*   *Investor*

Stage I: Preparation

You prepare for wealth creation by setting your vision and then entering the Power Matrix to identify your gifts, talents, and powers that you can develop into competencies for creating wealth. You recognize the stages and time frame of the

> *The problem is always the frame, and never the person.*

process and where you are in the stages. You start with your job to add value and to increase your income. With your finances you begin to plan and budget, save to build capital. You use frugality to get out of debt and begin saving in a serious way. You establish your beliefs, decisions, and principles for wealth creation.

The meaningful performances of wealth creation in this stage include: planning, budgeting, saving, frugality, self-investment in your learning, creativity, and self-actualization. One of the fascinating discoveries from Blotnick's twenty-year longitudinal study was that "almost none of the people we studied became rich doing the thing they started out to do." (p. 70). Isn't that incredible!? It always changed. Sometimes only moderately, sometimes radically. But it always changed. It did for me and I bet it will for you, and probably several times. And if that's the case, then what do you need in order to start where you are right now realizing that both you and your direction will shift and change over the years? The answer is obvious: *it requires flexibility.* Lots of flexibility! It requires that you will need to keep learning, developing, and planning as you go without demanding that you have it all figured out before you begin. In other words, you will keep inventing it as you go. (Chapters 3-5)

Stage II: Singularity

Here you enter the Self Matrix to engage in a talent search to find your singularity. You give yourself to your own self-investment in your learnings about what you are best able to do, your passions, your potentials, your creativity, etc.

Then by yourself, or with a mentor and/or coach, you identify and develop a singularity of your passion, potential, and profit. *Your potential* refers to what can you do and contribute. What value can you add? *Your passion* refers to what you care about, believe in, and enjoy. And *your profit* refers to what real-world job or business will enable you to live your passion.

Your singularity is the interface of your skills, interests, abilities, your passions with a market in which you can create a viable business. Here learning with persistence and resilience will eventually enable you to identify and make a commitment to your singularity. And when you have that, you have your direction for wealth creation.

The meaningful performances at this stage include: increasing your income, engaging in a talent search to discover your gifts, talents, and potentials for your singularity, making a decision and commitment about your direction, and establishing your identify as a wealth creator.

It all begins with evaluating, studying, and preparing your wealth creating states and skills. It requires acquiring your first level knowledge about finances and work. In this you are first learning the game— the rules of the financial and business games and how to play these games for fun and profit.

In his book *Creating Wealth*, Robert Allen says that this stage is like developing a booster rocket, like a Titan, so that you can blast off into the orbit of money making money for you. You will need a mechanism, an economic engine, that's powerful enough to do that. That's why you'll need a singularity that has passion at its heart. (Chapters 6-8)

Stage III: Collaborations
In this stage, you enter into the *Others Matrix* to find and develop the relationship and social skills so that you can find those who you want to be on your wealth creation team. Because wealth is created with and through others, wealth creation is a collaborative phenomenon. *No one gets wealthy alone.* Wealth is best created with partners, colleagues, and a team of people. You make them wealthy as they make you wealthy. And this requires that you be a good team player.

The meaningful performances at this stage involve developing the social and relational skills for getting the right people on the bus with you in your business, those who can and will support you. It involves developing the integrity to live your vision as you find and live your principles, it also involves learning to enjoy adding value to people and becoming a value-contributor to others.

Getting the right people on your bus means that you need team players to work with you. So, who do you need on your team? Who are the right people for you? Who are the wrong people?

> "The secret to success of the companies that become great and not just good is that they get the right people on the bus and the wrong people off the bus." (Jim Collins, *Good to Great*).
> "I only work with the best. I hire the best people from my competitors." (Donald Trump)

What relational and social skills for treating people well will you need to develop? How clear are you about your values and the values that you want in those you work with? Are your expectations high without being unrealistic? Wealth creation generally involves creative people who live on the edge, so set the standards high enough to keep them involved. Make people feel important. Do you know how to do that? Do you have a good sense of humor? Do you set people at ease in your presence? Do you give thought and time to speaking to them as persons? If people like you, that's half the battle. (Chapter 9)

Stage IV: Business Launch
The next matrix that you will enter is that of the *World Matrix* and specifically the domain or universe of business and your specific industry. With your singularity and team, you are now ready to set up your business as a wealth creation business. You are ready for the risk taking of entrepreneur-ing, of building your team, of branding, marketing, and selling with your unique selling point. Here also you will focus on meta-detailing your business expertise and using continuous learning to keep refining things.

The meaningful performances required at this stage include creating your business plan, your strategy, and steps required to make it work. You will need to turn your colleagues into business partners with whom you can create collaborative partnerships.

This stage may last for 5 or 10, even 15 years. If you have everything in place, then it's just a matter of time. And whether it requires three years or twenty, the wealth creation states you'll need are patience, persistence, and commitment. If you don't do this, then your game plan can easily be sabotaged and defeated by impatience and "get rich quick" thinking.

In this stage you will want to concentrate your forces and energies (skills, talents, focus) on one thing—your singularity. Focus on the expert skills crucial for success in your field and market. This is not the stage to diversify, it is the time to concentrate. Concentrate on becoming an expert, investing yourself fully, and increasing the value of what you do. Find your passion and fall in love with it—live, breathe, and nurture it.

As you follow the wealth creation principles in this stage, it's important also to invest only and always in "assets" (things that put money in your pockets) rather than in "liabilities" (things that demand that you pull money out of your pockets). (Chapter 10)

Stage V: Business Development
One of the worlds within the World Matrix is the world of business. So in this stage you systematize your business so that it has a life of its own and can operate without you. Doing that means that you will be making money even when you sleep or are on holiday. How does that sound? In this stage you will be grooming colleagues as leaders and managers, and developing a committed supply line and customers. This stage requires a lot of financial intelligence about taxes, multiple sources of income, capitalization, etc.

The meaningful performances in this stage include: specifying your supply line, expanding your business and number of colleagues, continuing to develop your financial intelligence, developing multiple sources of income, and using persistence and patience to stay the course.

Once you have your business in place, you'll want to develop it to the place where it can run on its own. How will you build momentum of customers, supplies, employees, etc.? What systems will you set in place?

Your passive income, multiple sources of income, reduction of debt, frugality, investments, accumulated interest, etc., works to put you in the place where you are now *financially independent*. This is not a description of how much money you have, it's a description of the fact that you don't *have to* go to work to live. You are *independent* of depending on working for your basic life-style. Your money now works for you giving you the lifestyle you want and the freedom to explore, contribute, and be according to your personal values and visions.

It began with the initial stage where you developed a plan, put your plan into action, and took the effective actions, day after day, week after week, year after year. Over the years of the inner game stage, you developed the mechanisms that has now gotten your wealth off the ground. With that, your money has begun to experience an accelerated growth. During years five to fifteen you automatize the processes so that the money works for you. (Chapter 10)

Stage VI: Investment
Throughout the first stages, you work for money. Now in this stage, money begins working *for* you. In fact, the day that money begins working for you is the day you move from employee and/or self-employed to owning a business or operating as an investor. You have now moved to the right side of the Cashflow Quadrants.

In this stage, you have made it to financial independence. You have become wealthy. Now you shift to a different mode—one of growing and maintaining the wealth you have created. Having becoming financially independent, perhaps even abundantly wealthy, the time will come to jettison all of your debts, consolidate your financial resources, diversity your savings and investments, and shift to thinking in terms of safety and protection. This will enable you to let the money protect you in the remaining years.

The *World Matrix* for this stage involves yet another "world"— the domain of investment. In this stage you use your learning and creativity to discover where and how to invest for a good return on your investment. You learn how to make investment meaningful, ethical, and a peak experience. The meaningful performances in this stage include: identifying investments, and accessing courage and resilience for investing.

In this stage you need continual vigilance, increase in your business sense about the economy, finances, markets, trends, taxes, etc. Becoming *business smart* is an essential part of long-term wealth building. Build systems and businesses that have a life of their own, that contribute to the world, that enrich people, and that bring in money while you are not at work, even when you are on holiday.

Regarding investing in the stock market, Dent (1998) recommends using buy and hold strategies to stay invested in fundamental bull markets. His strategy is to build wealth by systematically investing in long-term trends (p. 284). He says that the risk in highly predictable markets is not being in the market, but being out of it. Machig and Behrends (1997) say that patience and compound interest are two key factors that are essential to building wealth, two factors that involve time and a longer-term perspective. These are a few sample ideas for this stage.

There is a set of skills involved in investing. While it sounds as simple as giving your money to someone—a stock broker, a real estate agent, a bank, etc., it is not. Lots of investments, maybe even most of them, do not get money to work for you. With many investments you can lose money and even lose all the money you created. (Chapter 14)

The Stages of Creating Wealth

Kinds of Wealth

Being	Doing	Having	Giving

Learn:
- Be Frugal — Begin Business
- Budget — Develop Expert Knowledge — Legacy prepared
- Eliminating Debt — Partner with others
- Save — Delegate
- Handling money — — Find Partners — Exit Strategy
    – Clarify Market — Invest in business
    Create valuable P/S. — Employees
    Find your Singularity —> Develop your Singularity
    Concentration efforts / money — Diversification
    – Selling
    – Marketing — Investing in the business.
    – Branding

Investing in Self — Develop financial intelligence — Business/ Leadership Intelligence

Search Stage	**Development**	**Success**	**Diversification**
1-5 years	3- 8 years	5-20 years	10– 40 years

Stage VII: Exit
How will you exit your business? What legacy will you leave with the money and wealth that you have created? What will happen to it when you end your career path and when you die? What then?

The final stage is that of your exit strategy. How do you transfer your business and investments so that you can leave a legacy that reflects your values and the mark that you make in the world.

The meaningful performances in this stage include: developing a plan for exiting the business and creating a legacy with your money and investments. In this stage you will plan how to use your money to leave the kind of legacy that will support the values and visions that you have lived for. The research shows that you can do great damage to our children, grandchildren, friends, and relatives if you do not *manage the transfer* of your wealth and decide on the legacy that you want to leave. Intelligence in handling this stage is equally called for as it is at the beginning of the process.

Wealth Creating Performances
Because there are different stages of wealth creation, *each stage requires a different strategy.* Each stage will require a different game plan for how to navigate the particular stage and therefore a different set of best states. (Chapters 11-13). The vision of building wealth and freeing yourself from working for money requires making a plan to navigate your pathway until you reach financial independence. In the process you will need to develop your financial intelligence and integrity as well as develop a discipline in following-through in handling your money.

Because creating wealth involves steps and stages that occurs over time, patience is required. Lots of patience—even the patience to learn how to become patient! Use the "Wealth in a Decade" frame of mind. This will enable you to create a wealth orientation that will become your life style. And doing that will bring about another shift. You will move your focus from *the end product* (making lots of money) to enjoying *the process* (creating value that makes a difference). When you make this shift, you refocus on knowing and learning how to enjoy this day and every activity and feeling and being richer in your being, thinking, emoting, and doing. Paradoxically, this makes your contributions more valuable.

Blotnick's research of those who wanted to become rich but did not showed that "the shorter a time period people chose [about how long they expected it would take to become rich], the less likely they were to become rich." (p. 36). This corresponded with the attitude and state of overly wanting to get rich as if money is the end goal. If you want it too much, that very state of mind will interfere with the process and sabotage your efforts. Alan Anixter put it succinctly in these words:

> "Focusing on money prevents everything else from falling into place. Build a good business—the money will come along as a result."

My Personal Story
Once I finally began (and it took me a long time before I did), it took me six years to become financially independent and two years later I reached the first million mark in terms of equity. But if I count from the time that I felt fed up with living paycheck to paycheck, it took a lot longer. It took eight years to get sick and tired enough to make the decision to become financially independent.

When I found myself back to zero (in terms of savings and equity) in 1988, I decided I would never again let that happen. That's when I made the first decision. I made a decision to avoid being reduced to zero. It wasn't a big bold ferocious goal, but it was a beginning. At least it got me started.

At the time I was just getting by, making $15,000 to $20,000 a year as a counselor. Three years previously I had moved to Colorado spending half my time establishing a counseling business and half my time was involved in a ministry. The ministry provided $12,000, and the day my now ex-wife announced she was leaving to be with her supervisor, I was told to turn in my resignation. One event launched two losses. Given that our daughter was three years old, I made a decision to do everything within my powers to get custody. And after two years and enriching a layer to the tune of twelve thousand dollars as he managed (and sometimes perpetuated) the fight, I won custody.

By 1988 I had a grant total of $500 to my name. In the meantime, I bought a house in town and moved my office from the second floor of a professional office building in a bank to the house. Doing that transferred the money that I was spending for renting the office to invest in a larger home—the house in which I created my office. And that allowed me to be "home" and just one block from the elementary school for my daughter, Jessica. In fact, the school was on one end of the block and our home on the other.

How did I buy that house? I did so by doing two things: I rented the first house that I bought and had kept through the divorce and used the money that I pay for renting an office to buy the second house.

In making this move, I made another decision. Instead of selling the first house which I still owned even though all the equity had been taken out of it, I made it a rental property. I figured that because the mortgage was in my name, why give that up? Why not rent it and let someone else pay the mortgage? That decision turned my home (my first house) into an investment property and I thereby suddenly became a landlord. Yet with a greatly reduced salary, and no equity in the house, no bank would lend me money for a second house. Not the bank with whom I had the mortgage nor any other that I asked. I went through the asking application twelve times with twelve banks! No one would give me a mortgage. All of them considered me a very high risk! This led to realizing that to find a second house I would have to find a house that the owner would be willing to carry the loan for me.

Now I had been paying $350 to $400 for the counseling office and the conference room for trainings. So I decided to invest in real estate that I would own. I knew what I did *not* want— to throw that money "down the drain" for rent. It took me three months to find the new house that met my criteria: It had to be within city limits, it had to be close to a school, and it had to have room that would work for an office / training room. I eventually found a 1949 house on the corner of 7th and Orchard Streets. Years before its original two-car garage had been converted to a family room and another two-car garage had been built on to the house. I hired a contractor to open those two rooms thereby giving me a large room the size of two large two-car garages (21 feet by 33 feet, approximately 7 by 11 meters). And I had room for 5 cars to park with more room across the street at the Art Center.

And best of all, the owner of the house agreed to carry the loan of $87,000. Of course, he agreed to do that at 10.5 percent interest. And with that I became a "landlord" and began my wealth creation process. It wasn't easy; it wasn't fast. But it was a beginning, one that I had initiated. (Eight years later I sold the house for $150,000).

Your Adventure in Creating Wealth
Now that you've finished this chapter, are you ready for your Wealth Coaching? Great.

Your next Wealth Creation task is to use the seven stages of wealth creation as a map and to locate where you are in your own journey. Get your *Inside-Out Wealth Creation Journal* and using the time-line in this chapter, draw it in your journal. Now identify when you began, where you are now, and where you want to be in one year, two years, five, ten, etc. Put a check mark and a date—and jot down what you did or are doing at those dates.

After you take some time to fill in the time-line of your wealth creation journey, sit back and reflect on it. What are you aware of as you think about wealth creation as a life-time adventure? How will this realization help you? As you do so, listen for and be sensitive to any thoughts "in the back of your mind" that might be limiting beliefs. Write them down. We will use them later.

End of Chapter Notes
1. See *Self-Actualization Psychology* (2008).

2. See the book, *The Matrix Model* (2003) for a full presentation of the entire model, how it is constructed as a systems model about human thinking, feeling, acting, and relating and how to use it. Also see Chapter 15 where there is a short description of the Matrix Model and your ten-year wealth creation plan.

3. See *Winning the Inner Game* (2007) a book that uses the idea of "frames" and "games" to simplify the Meta-States model.

4. Regarding human emotions: they are primarily and mostly derivative of our thoughts. As you think, so you feel. Emotions primarily reflect and record your meanings— they are the feel of the meanings that you create about something. Yet because of our mind-body-emotion system, we also respond to our emotions. That is, we have thoughts about our emotions and so once we have an emotional experience, that then becomes information back into the system. And so round and round it goes.

Chapter 3

WHY DO IT?

"Vision without systems thinking ends up painting lovely pictures of the future with no deep understanding of the forces that must be mastered to move from here to there."
  Peter Senge (*The Fifth Discipline,* p. 12)

"The secret of success is constancy of purpose."
  Benjamin Disraeli

"Life will pay any price you ask of it.
So, what do you ask of life? How big are your goals?"
  Tony Robbins

Why create wealth? Wealth creation begins with a desire. You have to want it. You have to choose it. It will not just happen. You have to set a direction, make a decision for it, focus your energies, and arrange your lifestyle so that you are aligned in moving forward to wealth creation. But why do that?
- What's your highest intention in seeking to create wealth?
- What's your purpose?

Actually, it not only takes desire, it takes something more. *It takes a strong and robust desire, one for the long haul, and one that will handle the ups and downs that will inevitably come.* And then, when you have a robust desire, that will give birth to a vision for creating wealth that will enable you to unleash the skills and capacities that are required for you to become financially independent.

So it all begins with desire. It begins because you want more fullness and richness in your life, more money that gives you more freedom, choice, and opportunities. Or perhaps you begin with the away-from desire: you *do not want* poverty, limitations, creditors, worry, working for money, being money-focused, etc.

Either way, *the journey starts with desire*— desire toward and/or desire away-from. It is this primary state that you will refine, sharpen, and frame for wealth in every dimension of human experience. To facilitate this, here are some vision questions, first the away-from desires and then the toward-desires. While we all have both sets of desires, most of us operate from a preferred style —we use the push of the away-from energies or we use the pull of the toward-desires.

Aversions:
- What do you want no more?
- From what do you move away from?
- What will you no longer tolerate?
- How will you feel about that?
- Does this create enough aversion and disgust for you to make a change?
- How will it affect you emotionally, personally, interpersonally, spiritually, etc.

Attractions:
- What do you want? Describe your desire. Are you ready to dream?
- Do you know how to dream? Do you have permission to dream?
- What is your dream and vision about creating financial independence?
- Have you turned your dream into a well-formed outcome?
- Why is this important to you?
- What are the positive values of the vision?
- How will you feel when you have that fully and completely and just the way you want it?
- How will it enrich you personally, interpersonally, and spiritually?

Getting Your Great Big *Why*

If you're going to create inside-out wealth, you will have to *create a great big why*—one big enough to propel your neurological energies. If your idea becomes a burning desire in you, all you need to do is let it grow up into a magnificent obsession as you keep testing the reality of your plan and checking its ecology. It will then be current and appropriate. It will then become a self-organizing process that will prepare you to create the passion. This was perhaps the key that Napolean Hill emphasized in his books on creating wealth:

> "Every man is what he is because of the dominating thoughts which he permits to occupy his mind. Thoughts which a man deliberately places in his own mind and encourages with sympathy, and with which he mixes any one or more of the emotions, constitute the motivating forces which direct and control every moment, act, and deed." (Hill, 1960, p. 53)

So, do you have a big enough why? Do you have and do you know your magnificent obsession? If you do not, do you know how to create *a big enough reason* for creating wealth? And why is this important? To generate sufficient motivation for the wealth creation journey and the lifestyle it will require.

Wealth Motivation

I have just brought up the subject of motivation. Did you notice? Yet in bringing up motivation, I'm not speaking about *the rah-rah! type of motivation* that is so common when it comes to wealth creation trainings and workshops. While that can arouse passions and create excitement, *rah-rah! motivation is not what is needed for the long-term.* And in fact, it will *not* work for the long-term. That type of motivation is too shallow, too superficial, and too distracting for the long-term stages of wealth creation. You can't sprint a marathon. You need a different kind of motivation—a different kind of energy.

What often happens with a great many people is that they become addicted to *the rah-rah!* type of motivation. Then as soon as everyday life outside the excitement of the coliseum kicks in, they struggle to persist. They then begin wondering, "What's wrong with me?" "I've lost the passion and excitement I felt at the 'Become a Millionaire Now' seminar." And they falsely assume, "If I don't feel like it, I can't do it." Their lack of an emotional high of excitement then causes them to stop as they then focus on their emotional state. Yet the actual problem in this case is *the emotional high addiction* itself.

What's needed is another other type of motivation than *the rah-rah!* type that pounds the chest and walks across hot coals. In fact, *when a strong passionate desire grows up, it becomes an intention, a focus, a direction, and a purpose that you can take with you wherever you go.* You can then take it with you as your basic attitude or mental disposition. In other words, it grows up from a primary state of an emotional excitement into a meta-state of an attitude and disposition. Inside this more complex state the emotional engine is still there, but above and beyond that innate excitement is a more grown-up orientation—*an intention* that governs your consciousness. It is an intention that orders your energies and focus. And this brings us to the subject of intentionality.[1]

Intentional Motivation
Years ago I introduced in Neuro-Semantics Rollo May's two-fold distinction of consciousness: intention and attention. These two facets of consciousness make up the faculty that we call "will." *Attention* is what is *on your mind*. It is what you are aware of, thinking about, and focused on. To identify your attentions, notice what you are representing on the screen or movie of your mind. To identify the flow of your attentions during any given day, notice what gets your attention, grabs your attention, and what interrupts your attention. This is the world of attentions.

Yet the world of attentions is the world that animals, infants, and small children live in. *They live attentionally.* Now the funny thing about the world of attentions, the more you have, the more likely you are to be labeled with ADD. But of course, that's the joke—*there is no deficiency of attentions in Attention Deficit Disorder.* The problem is that there are too many attentions! And they are wildly out of control.

> *"Energy flows where attention goes as determined by intention."*

Actually, the problem with ADD is a deficient of intention. If I was in charge of the Department of Acronyms, I would relabel ADD and call it IDD (Intention Deficient Disorder). After all, the problem is that there's not enough intention. And what intention there is, it is not strong enough to carry one forward. We label someone as having ADD when they are in a context of needing to study grammar and they really do not want to. They want to play Playstation 3 or a computer game. We use the ADD label for the person who needs to pay attention to receipts, bills, accounting, etc. when the person's consciousness keeps shifting to the beach, going for a walk in the mountains, or going to the movies.

For the majority of people the problem isn't attention deficit, it is *intention deficit.* They do not *want* to do the things that they *need* to do, that some context requires to be done. It is important, but it does not *feel* important. It feels boring, tedious, uninteresting, undesirable.

Intention is not what is "on our mind." *Intention refers to what is in the back of the mind.* It is what we "know" at some level of awareness or knowledge we need to do, should do, that would be important to do, and that we "intend" to do. We do intend to do it. It is our intention to eat healthily, to exercise regularly, to clean our desk, to keep our bills paid on time, and so on. But then other things grab our attention, and off we go with the result that we forget what we intended to do.

> **The Intentionality Principle**
> *Wealth is created through the ability to weigh alternatives and make an informed decision and stay with it. Wealth is built through vison, well-formed outcomes, empowering decisions, becoming decisive, and the ability to stay with the decisions.*

Good intentions, poor follow-through. Good intentions, but not enough energy or motivation to get you to do what you know to do. What's the problem? Emotional motivation? Well, that can help ... for awhile. Then when the emotional high leaves, you're back at the same place.

So what is the solution to this merry-go-round of plans, intentions, and attentions? *It is to energize your intentions and then robustly connect them to your attentions so that your attentions do service to your highest intentions.* Then you will begin to live intentionally rather than attentionally. And this is truly the human way to live—from your highest intentions rather than your moment-to-moment attentions. Then you live purposefully from what you decide you will do rather than what you feel like doing at any given moment.

It is intentionality that can endow your passions with a strong laser-beam focus and concentration so that you develop a magnificent obsession and let it direct your way of being in the world. This is where wealth creation begins. It begins as you intentionally choose your values, your dreams, and the life that you way to live.

It is intentionality also by which you can set up *a self-organizing attractor* in your mind-body system. This means that as you intentionally set your direction and values. Then the frames you set establish the self-organizing process. That is, your beliefs about these values and directions then become self-fulfilling prophecies. And as values, they are attractors of the experiences, people, ideas, and emotions that correspond to them. You see the world in terms of these intentions.

So the ability to step up to your highest intentions and take an intentional stance enables you to operate from the values that you deem valuable. For example, you can now choose to operate from abundance, cooperation, and integrity. You can choose to operate from seeing and seizing opportunities. You can choose to operate from creating and living your dream. You can choose to live by whatever values you set as your intentions.

In Neuro-Semantics we have a specific pattern designed to enable you to *take an intentional stance,* to specify your highest intentions and to then connect them to your everyday activities. That pattern is reproduced here to give you a chance to get your attentions to do service for your highest intentions.

Intentionality Pattern

To work through this process, you can start with any work-related activity that you perform as part of your plan for creating wealth. You can choose something very positive or very negative. It doesn't matter, just as long as it is important to you. That is, you *know* it is important, it just *doesn't feel* that way and especially when you need to do it. What are some of the tasks that you engage in as part of your wealth building process? What do you need to do in order to succeed? When you have identified one, use that activity as a reference point to explore your higher intentions.

After you have identified some activity to explore, answer these

questions:
> How is that activity important to you? How is it valuable? How is it meaningful? In what way? What else is important about that?

The process begins with these questions, so be sure to answer them. Don't worry about problems of doing it, focus simply on one thing—*identifying the value of the activity.* Is the activity valuable in getting you want you ultimately want?

Now holding that value in mind—how it is important—ask the *"Why* is it important?" question seven more times, or as many times as you need to. Each time you do this, you move up a meta-level. Hold that as the next level value, and ask the question again.
> "So this activity is important to you because of these things. And how is this important to you? What's important by having this?"

If you're doing this by yourself, then write down the value on a piece of paper, then as you sit back and look at it. Now ask the intention question again:
> "What is important about that outcome? And what's even more important than that? And when you get that fully and completely and in just the way you want it, what's even more important?"

Continue to do this until you flush out and detect all of the higher values that you have about that in the back of your mind.

Eventually you will get to the top. How will you know? You will either begin looping around a couple of the values, re-stating it again and again. Or you'll go blank and there'll be nothing more. Or you will say or have the sense, "That's it." "There's nothing else. It is just this."

When you get there, simply imagine stepping into the higher value state or states of importance so that you feel them fully. Just welcome in the good feelings that these meanings invite, and just be with those higher level feelings for a bit. Do you like that? Let those feelings grow and intensify as you recognize that this is your highest intention. This is what you are all about... isn't it? Enjoy this awareness. Accessing this state is just like accessing any state, as you think about it, represent it, welcome it into your body and be with that feeling.[2]

Now that you are in this higher state and frame of mind, apply it to the first state.

> "Having these higher feelings in mind... fully... imagine this intentional stance getting into your eyes, into your body, into your way of being in the world and imagine moving out into life tomorrow with them... and as you do ... and as you engage in that work-related activity that's part of your wealth creation plan, notice how the higher frames transforms it... And take all of this into tomorrow and into all of your tomorrows ..."

When you do this you are meta-stating your attentions with your highest intentions. You are linking the two so that in your everyday attentions, you don't forget your reasons why, your highest intentions.

> **Meta-Stating:** The process of bringing one state to another to create a new and more complex state, so *joy* to *learning* creates the state of *joyful learning*.

As you now check this out, if it is ecological for you—if it fits into all the dimensions of your life, then commission your executive mind to take ownership of this. Do that by answering this question:

> "There's a part of your mind that makes decisions, that chooses the pathway that you want to go, will that highest executive part of your mind take full responsibility to "be of this mind" about this activity and to remind you to see the world this way?"

If you need any other resources, then simply access that resource and integrate it into your new state. Would you like to bring any other resource to this intentional stance? Would playfulness enrich it? Persistent? Passion? Etc.

Intentionality as Attitude
I'd recommend you run the intentionality pattern on five to seven activities that you know are important to you, yet which you really struggle to implement. Do this that many times and you will begin to find a pattern— you will keep rising up to a group of values that are really important to you (these are your highest valued meta-states). Then do the same thing with five to seven activities that you already know and *feel* as important.

Another discovery you will make from this will be how your highest felt values—values that excite you and feel passionate about—become incorporated as your attitudes. *They become your mental frames of mind.* This is critical because if your frames

> Suze Orman (1999) says that regarding values and priority of what's important as: "People first, then money, then things."

of mind are not intimately connected with your everyday activities, your life will be incongruent and out-of-alignment with your highest values. And when that happens, you'll not feel whole, not feel "right," and not experience the power of personal congruency.

What will solve this? The solution is to repeatedly run the intentionality process. Do that and you will begin to create the linkage again and again between your highest intentions and your lifestyle. And do it enough, eventually you will find it easy and natural to connect your highest intentions to your everyday actions. This will empower your attitude so that it is super-charged, that is, highly robust and powerful. And then you will have solved the motivation problem. You will then have the motivation to carry through. The step after that is making sure your intentions inform your decisions.

From Intentionality to Decision
Once you integrate your passionate motives (values) as your inner motivation, you will be able to make empowering decisions and thereby be the architect to your way of life. You will be able to make the decision to become a wealth creator, to create wealth, and the hundreds of supporting decisions that will help to make this real. Actually, this is a critical facet of a healthy wealth creation strategy. To create wealth you will have to make hundreds, if not thousands, of smaller decisions about how you will actualize your strategic plans. And such enhancing decisions arise from the clarity of your values and criteria.

What is the relationship between your intentions and your decision? *Your overall decision is your intention and from it come all of your sub-decisions.* In the process of deciding, you engage in the two dimensions of thought known as attention and intention.

> You *intend* a goal, outcome, passion, direction, purpose.
> You *attend* to it until you realize it in your life.

Now energy flows where attention goes, does it not? Yes, of course, what you attend to elicits your mental and emotional energies. And energy can now flow where attention goes as you determine it by your highest intentions. This means you can now use this psychological dynamic to empower yourself to align all of your daily attentions to your highest intentions of wealth creation.

What is the way to gain mastery over procrastination? It is through intentional decisiveness. Decisiveness is the key. It is the power to *cut* (de-cision) your path, to divide the Red Sea before you that's in your way and move forward to your promised land. And what creates decisiveness? The simplest of things— yes and no. To decide on your goal, to say *yes* to it, you have to say *no* to everything that gets in the way or distracts you from it.

The word "decision" literally refers to this cutting process. *De-cision* refers "to cut" one away "from" another. And you do this by the using the two knives (yes and no) as scissors by which you can cut off the alternatives from the chosen pathway.

Decisiveness gives you a sense of mission allowing you to think, feel, and act purposefully. From a committed decision comes a vitality of mind-and-emotion to see opportunities. After all, it takes strength of heart to see the difficult tasks ahead and to face them head-on. When you make a hard decision, you will be able to say *Yes* and *No* to choices, and to follow through.

Decisiveness arises from the strength of your intentionality. And it shows up as you choose your plan and choose to stay with it through thick and thin. Napolean Hill described the role of making decisions and its relationship to creating wealth:

> "Analysis of several hundred people who had accumulated fortunes well beyond the million-dollar mark disclosed the fact that every one of them had the habit of reaching decisions promptly, and of changing these decisions slowly, if, and when they were changed. People who fail to accumulate money, *without exception,* have the habit of reaching decisions, if at all, very *slowly,* and of *changing these decisions quickly and often."* (p. 139)

Thomas Stanley described the value of having a clear and focused intention relating it to having goals in whatever we do:

"The students who get the most out of their formal education are those who fully realize the specific value of what they are studying. They are the ones who have the least difficulty earning their degrees and who get the most out of their programs. ... If you are without goals, college may be a nightmare. The earlier in life you determine what you really want to do, really want to become, the easier and more purposeful your training will be." (Stanley, 2000, pp. 208, 209)

> "Someone who has money as their goal is actually wandering around blinded— they have no way to tell which direction is right, for them."
> *Oscar Dystel*
> Former Chairman and CEO, Bantam Books

The bottom line is this: *It takes a powerful intention to mobilize your potentials and energies.* Without a powerful intention, then your attention drifts to whatever is before you. Without a powerful intention you will end up watching the clock, spending your time wishing and wanting to be somewhere else doing something else. Without a powerful intention, it is hard, if not impossible, to be present and fully engaged in what you are doing. And without a powerful intention you have no higher frame of mind that enables you to see opportunities and take advantage of them.

A Clean Intention

I doubt that there will be any question with developing a powerful and focused intention, but the next piece, developing *a clean intention,* this may evoke questions and doubts. Why do you need a clean intention for your wealth creation? Because if your motive is not clean—if it is contaminated by greed, fear, competition, revenge, needing to prove your value, and so on— that kind of intention and motive will undermine the inside-out wealth creation process.

This is what I learned from the many, many case studies that Scrully Blotnick (1980) extensively described. In that longitudinal study, he discovered that people who have almost any focus and motive other than enjoying their work and the difference it makes for others, inevitably sabotages their ability to get rich. As he repeatedly asked his millionaires, multi-millionaires, and want-to-be-millionaires, "Why do you want to get rich?" those who wanted to "show them," gain acceptance, or compete against someone almost always ended up defeating themselves (p. 136, and chapter 10).

That's why it is essential to make sure that your *reasons why* — your intentions—for creating wealth are clean and uncontaminated by negative emotions and negative motives. We'll revisit this in Part III when we explore the negative states that undermine the wealth creation ability.

> **The Planning Principle:** *Wealth is created by developing a plan for how to manage finances, a plan for focusing attention on skills, interests, passions, and talents in adding value.*

Your Decisive Intentionality

After you use the intentionality pattern a number of times (and I recommend five to ten times), write your intentions for wealth creation down on a piece of paper. What is your highest and biggest intention? What are some of your other high intentions? Now begin to write down some of the practical actions that you have to do to begin the process. What do you need to do now? What do you have to do today, this week, this month, to begin your wealth creation process? Here are some ideas that might prompt your thinking as you create your list:

    __ Read one chapter of this book each day.
    __ Record all of my expenses to see where my money goes.
    __ Create a budget for my expenses.
    __ Clean my desk and set up a way to save receipts.
    __ Create a plan for controlling my spending.
    __ Ask myself, "Is this the best way to do this?"
    __ Identify three ways to improve the quality of my work.
    __ Use frugality to control my spending.
    __ Contact three people to interview about X.
    __ Create a system for keeping receipts in a manageable form.

Once you have a list of actual behaviors to do, you have moved to a choice point. Now you are at the unique place where you can make an empowering decision. Will you do these things or not? Will you make an empowering decision to take action, invest your time and effort, or not?

From Decisive Intention to Planning

While it might seem that making these empowering decisions completes the process, it does not. You're not yet done. Once you have your *why*— your intention, and have made a decision about the specific things you are going to have to do, you still have to create a roadmap about how you will turn your dreams, goals, outcomes, and decisions into reality. Creating your specific roadmap is what planning is all about and it comes after the decision and intention. It is the planning process that makes your *why* real.

If you want to navigate the pathway of wealth you will need your own individualized plan that details how you will get there. What knowledge of the field of finances enables you to build an accurate, useful, practical, and workable map? There's an almost magical quality in planning. So as you first set your outcome for creating wealth, you now need to identify the details for your wealth creation plan.

Planning enables you to establish a direction for your hopes and dreams. Planning empowers your decision making and prioritizing puts some real teeth into your dreams. Planning clarifies the big picture, gives precision to your unifying theme, organizes your thinking, and directionalizes your attention. Planning crystallizes your desire so that you can put it into action.

This means committing your ideas and decisions and intentions to paper. It means creating a written plan. And once you have that, you can then use it as your blueprint, your business plan, and your checklist. Then you can consult it weekly and refresh it from time to time as you update it. Using meanings, principles and beliefs about wealth that support you, your plans will include how to reality-test your progress and how to set up milestones for measuring how you are progressing.

If you are still tempted to dismiss planning as too simple, here are two quotations about the importance of planning:
> "Creating wealth is simple. Yet most people never build it because they have holes in their financial foundations. These can be found in the form of internal values and belief conflicts, as well as poor plans that virtually guarantee financial failure." (Anthony Robbins, p. 456)
> "I believe that anyone who has a plan, self-discipline, investment knowledge, and a bit of patience can be wealthy." (Machtig, p. 2)

Ken Barlett's Planning Questions

I met Ken Barlett in 1999 with my first wealth creation training in New York city. When I met Ken he was a NLP counselor whose expertise was in career and financial counseling. And Ken had learned the importance of financial planning the hard way—by losing a fortune and discovering the importance of handling money well. Having inherited a lot of money and not knowing the value of a dollar, it only took him a few years to blow it all.

Afterwards, returning to university and using NLP as his model, Ken created a set of questions as central to his work with clients who wanted to create wealth. Here are his seven questions:

1) Do you have a plan?
2) Do you know how to make a plan?
3) Do you know how to stick to your plan?
4) Do you know how to keep refining your plan?
5) Are you willing to make and follow a plan?
6) Are you willing to do anything it takes and to do it well?
7) Do you know how to inspire yourself so that you will follow your plan?

Let's apply this to your wealth creation. Which of the following aspects of creating wealth do you need to create a plan so that you can effectively handle these facets?

- Developing your talents and skills for creating the value that will make money.
- Identifying your potentials and passions.
- Connecting your competencies with a business or need.
- Rendering useful and valuable services.
- Budgeting the money you now have to handle.
- Saving in a regular and methodical way.
- Getting out of debt.
- Investing in your own development.
- Business development.
- Marketing and selling.
- Investing in your business or the business of another.

> **Ken Barlett's Questions
> for your Wealth Business Plan:**
>
> 1) Do you have a plan?
> 2) Do you know how to make a plan?
> 3) Do you know how to stick to your plan?
> 4) Do you know how to keep refining your plan?
> 5) Are you willing to make and follow a plan?
> 6) Are you willing to do anything it takes and to do it well?
> 7) Do you know how to inspire yourself so that you will follow your plan?

My Personal Story

When I began, my motives and intentions were simple and low: to *not* be reduced to zero again. As time when on, I raised my intention: To create financial stability. After a few more years I raised my intention again: To build financial value so that I can create the independence to do what I want to do. Fast forward a few more years and my intentions grew to new heights and levels: To create enough wealth so that I can invest in things that I care about, that make a difference, in the quality of life for people using Neuro-Semantics, to build a trust fund of a million dollars for NLP research, to build a twelve-million dollar trust fund to take over an inner city school and demonstrate what we can do with a school of NLP teachers, to create a dozen ten-million dollar trust funds to establish Neuro-Semantic Chairs at ten Universities.

You can see from this that as my intentions developed, they became less centered on me and my lifestyle and more on the value that I could create and leave that would make a difference in the world and leave a positive legacy. And as the intentions got higher, thinking about making money and investing my time and effort in making money increasingly became what it is—a tool for being able to do things, to extend my powers and influence, and to fulfil values and dreams important to me. I found my big enough *why*.

Today I'm still very intentional in my wealth creation strategies. While I have several books that are best sellers in the field of NLP, I am still working and planning to write a best seller that will get onto the New York Times best seller list. So I continue to write on a daily basis as well as study writing. I also know that I can do so much more *with others* than alone, so I work to support Neuro-Semantics and Meta-Coach communities.

Your Adventure in Creating Wealth
Coaching time! Okay, so *why* do it? *Why* will you engage in the process of creating wealth? Do you have a big enough and clean enough reason for creating wealth? If not then spend time working through the intentionality pattern. Run that pattern ten times during this coming week in order to clarify your highest intentions and values.

Once you have that, begin to write out a list of your first decisions for your wealth creation plan. You can write them in your *Wealth Journal* or in the *Inside-Out Wealth Creation Plan* (chapter 15).

Are you expecting to have a *rah-rah!* motivation of excitement every day in all of your stages of wealth creation? Is your motivation up and down, on and off? Are you ready to develop an attitude of motivation that you can take with you for the rest of your life?

End of Chapter Notes
1. For more about motivation, see *Motivation: How to be a Positive Force in a Negative World* (1987).

2. Accessing a state refers to a basic NLP process. We do this all of the time, but most people do not do it intentionally and consciously. The process essentially involves identify the thoughts, ideas, and physiology that correspond to a state. For a description see *MovieMind* (2003) or *User's Manual for the Brain, Volume I* (1999).

Chapter 4

WHAT WILL IT MEAN?

"All wealth begins in the mind"
*"Every time he took the thought to bed with him,
he got up with it in the morning,
and he took it with him everywhere he went."*
Napoleon Hill (p. 96)

*"The secret of success in life
is for a man to be ready for his opportunity when it comes."*
Benjamin Disraeli

To be a wealth creator and to create wealth for yourself and others requires that you know what wealth is and is not, how it is created, and its relationship to money. You also need to have some rich and robust meanings about all of the wealth creation facets—creating value in a economic market with others that builds or supports a business.
- So what is wealth?
- What are the dimensions of wealth?
- What is money and how does it relate to wealth?
- What does it mean to create, own, have, and experience financial wealth?
- What are the pathologies that are connected to wealth and/or money?

Confusing Money with Wealth

To clear the air right from the start, *money is not wealth.* Money is one facet of wealth, and is the primary way that we measure *financial* wealth, but in itself, it is not wealth. Wealth is something other than money. So, what is money and what is wealth?

"Money" refers to the currency within any economy—the paper and coins that a government produces as symbols of value. Of course, this means that almost every time you cross a border and enter into another country, the "money" you bring with you ceases to be "money" there. On one side of the border, it is money; on the other side, it is not. It doesn't count there as useable currency. What is recognized and acknowledged as "money" is relative to the country and the government that issues the particular denominations of dollars, pounds, euros, pacos, deutch marks, rubles, yens, etc. "Money" is what we say is money.

It only takes a brief reflection about this to realize that "money" actually is not a real thing. It is does not actually exist "out there" apart from validating contexts. So what exists out there? Paper and coins, credit cards, and checks—these are the things that exist in the real world that we think of as money (we consider money, we deem money), but these are just symbols. So what is money?

> ***Money is a shared agreement within a social and political context, a way of thinking and feeling about how we exchange the value of our time, energy, and knowledge.***

Suppose I work for an hour designing a car, you work an hour building the car, another works an hour fixing a car, washing a car, selling a car, and so on, how do we measure *the value of the hour* that each person spends? We measure the *hour* that each person spends, along with the *knowledge and skills,* the *experience*, and so on that we use as we invest ourselves (our minds, emotions, actions, etc.) by an amount of money we receive for the given activity. So "money" represents how we value something. The more the product, service, or experience is valued (and by more people), the more "money" we can receive for it. Money is the scorecard that we use to measure the quality of knowledge and the quantity of time and effort we invested.

The term "money" itself is not an empirical term, it is a meta-term. It does not refer to an empirical see, hear, feel, smell, or taste reality. It refers to something you cannot see—something in your mind—*the value* you attribute to something in your mind. It refers to the meaning that you attribute to the value of something.

If this seems confusing, good! It is for most people when they first encounter this. It was for me. In fact, it took quite awhile for me to fully get my head around this. And that's because this refers to the neuro-semantic structure of "money." So here we go.

Figure 4:1

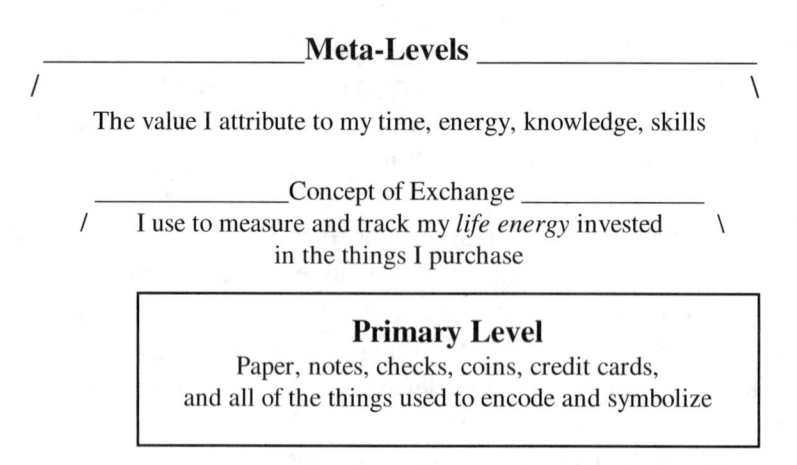

```
_____Meta-Levels_____
/                                              \
     The value I attribute to my time, energy, knowledge, skills

              _____Concept of Exchange_____
     /         I use to measure and track my life energy invested    \
                         in the things I purchase

              ┌─────────────────────────────────────────┐
              │             Primary Level                │
              │  Paper, notes, checks, coins, credit cards, │
              │ and all of the things used to encode and symbolize │
              └─────────────────────────────────────────┘
```

"Money" is the concrete thing that we for measuring and exchanging value—the value of the things that we invest our life energies into, the things that we do, know, and create. If that's what money is and what we use it for, this enables us now to ask several questions that will open new possibilities for wealth creation:
- How much value can I create with my time and energies?
- How much is my knowledge worth?
- How much is the service that I know how to deliver regarding X worth?
- What can I exchange my skills, knowledge, and expertise for money?

Because what counts for "money" differs between countries and cultures, *money is a shared cultural and political reality.* Different cultures also attribute different meanings and beliefs about exchange, time, skills, knowledge, and experiences. How you or any given family, religion, or culture frames these *exchanges* (that we measure by money), and the emotions it creates, determines how people think and feel about money. And if money is not real, then this exposes the myth that "there's only so much to go around." We humans can and do *invent* more money, more value, more wealth all the time. It happens every day. Just watch the stock markets or the price of oil and other commodities. How much money something "costs" can go up and down radically in minutes. That's because *the value of the money lies in the minds of people,* not in the money itself.

> "Money is something we choose to trade our life energy for."
> Dominguez (p. 54)

Different beliefs about money depends on the meanings we give to our investment of time, energy, mind, knowledge, care, emotion, etc. What do you believe about these things? Is your time "money?" Are your ideas and knowledge "money?" What about the care and attention you give to someone? Is that valuable? How much is that worth? What do you believe about products and services that you and others create, sell, and/or exchange? What about your reputation? Your name?

No wonder the process of identifying the meaning of money is complex. Money can mean so many things. It also can mean different things at different levels. So as you move up the levels to the higher (or meta) levels, the meanings that you create can become quite expansive. The meanings you ascribe to all of these different facets of money semantically load money. And with that, money gets connected to psychological categories such as power, status, love, control, freedom, etc.

- How much does this open up your understanding of money and finances?
- What do you now know or feel about money?
- How will this influence you in your own creation of wealth?
- Does this make money seem more or less important to you?
- What else does it open up for you?

The Neuro-Semantics of Wealth

About the Matrix, Morpheus asked Neo, "Do you want to know what *it* is?" So about money and about wealth, you have to know what *it* is if you want to experience wealth fully. For a healthy inside-out wealth, it is important to create a holistic and compelling definition of "wealth." Then you can more easily take the necessary and effective actions to make it real in your life. Do you know what *wealth* is?

Start with any one or more of the following sentence stems, put it at the top of a sheet of paper and write five to ten completions.
"*I know I will be wealthy when ...*"
"*True wealth for me is...*"
"*The wealth that I want and will pursue is ..*"

Don't skip this exercise! Okay, how did that go? Did you do it? How do *you* define wealth? How do you *want* to define it so that you have a rich and robust understanding of wealth so that you find it attractive, desirable, compelling, holistic, and ecological?

And why go through the trouble of mapping the meaning of wealth? Mostly so that you can be clear about what it is that you want to create and can know what it is that you will give yourself to. Here are some possibilities of how to define "wealth."

1) Income.
The first thing that most of us think about when we define wealth is income—salary. In this perspective, you define wealth in terms of having a high income or lots of perks with your income, bonuses, and/or the compensation package that comes with your job. So, if you define it in terms of income, how much do you need to make or to accumulate before you can think of yourself "wealthy" or "financially independent?"

2) Accumulation: net worth and savings.
Another place that we typically begin in defining wealth is to define it in terms of our net worth. How much money, income, savings, investments, equity do you want or need in order to be or to feel "wealthy?" How much do you have to have?

Stanley and Danko (1996) offer the following formula for determining *wealth* and use it to determine if you are wealthy:
> "Multiply your age times your realized pretax annual household incomes from all sources except inheritances. Divide by ten. This, less any inherited wealth, is what your *net worth* should be." (p. 13)

Age X Annual Income ÷ 10

Examples: (30) X $30,000 = $900,000   ÷ 10 = $90,000
(40) X $40,000 = $1,600,000   ÷ 10 = $160,000
(50) X $50,000 = $2,600,000   ÷ 10 = $260,000

From this they set up two styles or categories of accumulating net worth and two groups of people— the PAWs and the UAWS:

PAW stands for *Prodigious Accumulator of Wealth.* PAWs are the builders of wealth. They save and so are the best at building net worth. In the study of first-generation rich millionaires, they typically have a minimum of four times the wealth accumulated.

UAW stands for *Under Accumulator of Wealth.* UAWs typically live above their means and emphasize consumption. They tend to de-emphasize many of the key factors that underlie wealth building (p. 15).

"Most people have it all wrong about wealth in America. Wealth is not the same as income. If you make a good income each year and spend it all, you are not getting wealthier. You are just living high. Wealth is what you accumulate, not what you spend." (p. 1)

3) *Stuff— possessions, toys, things.*
Another common choice for defining wealth is to define it in terms of the accumulation of certain possessions and/or luxury items—houses, cars, clothes, jewelry, etc. or in terms of experiences—exotic vacations, exclusive clubs and organizations, etc. If you define wealth in terms of stuff, how much stuff do you need? What stuff counts for you? Do you need two cars? Five? Do you need a vacation house? Do you need a hot tub?

4) *A sense of choice.*
Some people define and measure wealth in terms of the freedom of choice. Here wealth is about lifestyle and a sense of being in control of what you do and how you live your life. Wealth may now be defined as: "I am wealthy when I reach the point where my decision to go to work is *not* determined by financial needs." Machtig and Behrends speak about this in the following quotation, followed by one from Harry Dent:

"You are wealthy if you can take off from work to investigate a project that is important to you for non-financial reasons." (p. 9)

"Wealth is about giving yourself the freedom to choose the lifestyle that you want and to champion causes that you believe in." (p. 22)

5) *Time.*
Or how about this? What about measuring wealth in terms of time rather than dollars? Kiyosaki (2000) uses this definition when he asks, How many days can you live at your current standard of living?
> "Wealth is a person's ability to survive so many number of days forward. If I stopped working today, how long could I survive ... and maintain my lifestyle? (p. 73, also page 34)

6) *High effort–to–result ratio.*
What is wealth? George David, M.D. defines wealth as a relationship or ration between effort and results.
> "Wealth is when small efforts produce large results; poverty is when large efforts produce small results."

This fits with what Edward Gibbon wrote in 1814 in his *Memories*: "I am rich indeed, since my income is superior to my expenses, and my expense is equal to my wishes." If wealth is your inner sense of effectiveness and efficiency, how wealthy are you? If wealth is creating lots of results with minimal effort, what increases your wealth? Perhaps the next one.

7) *Creativity.*
You could measure wealth by the amount of rich creative ideas, perceptions that allow you to see opportunities and solve problems. We literally create wealth with new ideas—creative ideas that lead to new inventions and innovations. Big bucks is shelled out for new creative ideas. Whole companies are organized for this. This perspective defines wealth in terms of creativity. Then if you lost all of your money and possessions, it would be no big deal precisely because you have plenty more of creative ideas. This is Robert Allen's definition in the following:
> "Wealth is not money. Money is just the appearance of wealth. The form, but not the substance. Wealth is thoughts, not things. You can be wealthy without having lots of money. And you can be rich and not be wealthy. Now that may be a bit confusing, but it's true. Wealth is a state of mind—an attitude."

8) *Health and well-being.*
The word "wealth" comes from the older word, "weal," and means being

in a "sound, healthy or prosperous state, well-being." This corresponds to the dictionary definition of wealth as an "abundance of supplies, possessions, and resources." This means you could define wealth in terms of your resources for energy and vitality which gives you a resource for doing the things that you enjoy. You would then consider yourself wealthy when you have the health, energy, and vitality to live with a robust sense of well-being.

9) *Joy and enjoyment.*

You generally want more money so that you can enjoy certain things—possessions and experiences. And you do that so that you can have a state of joy. So you could now define wealth as joy, enjoyment, delight, and fun. A millionaire in the Stanley and Danko study said:

> "There are more people (employees) today working at jobs that they don't like. I'll tell you honestly that the successful man is a guy who works at a job, who likes his work, who can't wait to get up in the morning to get down to the office, and that's my criteria. And I've always been that way. I can't wait to get up and get down to the office and get my job under way." (p. 240)

After all, how wealthy are you if you are miserable all day long at work? How wealthy are you if you don't value your work or have fun doing it?

10) *Character and inner states.*

Wealth in this definition is *who you are*—your character, your sense of self, and your relationship with those you love. The next two quotes express this definition of wealth:

> "Tell your children that there are a lot of things more valuable than money: good health, longevity, happiness, a loving family, self-reliance, friends, reputation, respect, integrity, honesty, achievements. Money is icing on the cake of life. You don't ever have to cheat or steal, don't have to break the law or cheat on your taxes." (Stanley & Danko, 1996, p. 195)

Donald Trump:

> "My father's faith gave me unshakable confidence. It wasn't money that my father gave me; it was knowledge. It's much more important to be smart than right."

11) *Ease and comfort.*

A big reason most of us want more money, and a lifestyle of wealth, we see it as providing us a more comfortable lifestyle. This reminds me of the statement I've heard from many: "I've been rich and I've been poor; and I've had problems being both rich and poor. I prefer having problems with money than apart from money!" With sufficient money, you can hire out a lot of life's chores and especially the unpleasant chores. So perhaps your definition of wealth is, "I know I'll be wealthy when I can hire someone to cut my grass, or clean my house, etc."

12) Power.

Money has always been easily connected and linked to power and the reason is simple. With money you have the power (the ability) to get things, do things, go places, have others do things for you, etc. This explains why people can easily connect wealth with power and define wealth in terms of power—the power to buy, the power to have people jump at your command, the power to influence others, to contribute to causes, to have your ideas and beliefs published and broadcasted. "I know I'll be wealthy when I can get one person (ten, one hundred, one thousand, one million —pick your number) to share my belief in Y."

13) Etc.

How else could you measure wealth? Here are some additional choices that you might want to include in your wealth definition:
- Maximizing talents
- The legacy you get to leave
- Exchanging or bartering for something of value
- Enriching your knowledge
- Accessing rich emotional states

Given all of these possibilities, how do you want to expand your definition of wealth so that your definition and understanding of it is rich and expansive? What will you do want to add to your current understanding to expand your definition of wealth? Take time now to put together your wealth definition.

Good. Now let's test it. As you look over your new definition of what wealth is and how you will know that you are wealthy, does it include wealth of mind, ideas, emotion, lifestyle, relationship, heart, creativity, health, energy, motivation, passion, and so on?
What would you like to include in your definition of wealth to make it even richer? Does your definition attract you? Does it feel compelling to you? Is it something you want to attain?

Knowing what you are pursuing enables you to have *a clear target* for your aim. It also gives you something valuable and attractive. And for the great majority of people, money alone is not enough. Wealth is not about money, it is about your experiences which create money for you and the experiences that the money makes available for you.

Oh yes, there's one more thing about this process. Typically at this point in the Inside-Out Wealth trainings lots of people experience an "Aha!" moment. I have had people exclaim out loud in a state of utter surprise, "I'm already wealthy!" They came into the training feeling poor or desperate or unsettled in their financial state and suddenly discovered that they are wealthy, much wealthier than they ever knew. How about you?

The Psychology in Wealth
Let me now present the questions again:
- What does money *mean* to you?
- What do you believe about earning money, saving money, and spending money?
- What does this concept of money mean to you and how are those meanings governing and motivating how you act (perform) when it comes to money?

Given your ability to create meaning, you can create and endow money with far too much meaning. That is, you can *semantically load* money so that it becomes far too important, even insanely important to you. This was the point of an article in *Psychology Today* several years ago.

"For most people, money is never just money, a tool to accomplish some of life's goals. It is love, power, happiness, security, control, dependency, independence, freedom and more. Money is so loaded a symbol that to unload it—and *I believe that it must be unloaded to live in a fully rational and balanced relationship to money*—reaches deep into the human psyche. Usually, when the button of money is pressed, deeper issues emerge that have long been neglected." (January/February, *Psychology Today*, 1999, "Men, Women, & Money," by Olivia Mellan)

What meanings do you, consciously or unconsciously, give to money? Here's a checklist of common meanings that we give to money. Put a check by the following psychological states and values that currently are connected and associated with wealth for you:

Figure 4:2

Status	Security/ Safety	Being a Somebody
Achievement	Power	Independent
Opportunity	Fulfillment	Choices
Exchange	Self-Esteem	Selfish
Greedy	Ease	Danger
Happiness	Wholeness	Jealousy by others
Prestige	Personal Worth	Pleasure
Love	Desirability	Control
Freedom		

To *semantically load* money with these psychological states is to give money too much meaning—more meaning than it can bear. Overloading money with too much meaning then changes money so it works on you like a drug. "Money" becomes a psycho-active drug when your mood, happiness, peace of mind, etc. is *dependent* upon it. It then becomes an addiction.

"When I have money, I'm happy; when I don't, I'm worrisome, unhappy, miserable, a nobody, etc."

It is this semantic loading that then causes some people to over-value money, make it "the meaning of life," and trigger us for psycho-earning and psycho-spending. Then like psycho-eating[1], it becomes too addictive in your experience. Then you become "money-mad," greedy, insatiable, and like other addicts unable to control yourself with regard to your spending or working.

What's the solution? The solution is to give it the right amount of meaning. The solution is to accurately and appropriately define money and wealth—enough so that you recognize how it is important, and the degree of its importance, *and what it cannot do*. And when you do this, you set proper mental and emotional limits on money.

To develop a healthy and appropriate wealth creation plan, many people first have to *de-pleasure* money, things, and their definitions of wealth so that they are not so dominated by it. They need to de-load the semantic load so that they are not victims of psycho-earning or psycho-spending. Desperately needing money typically prevents you from effectively handling money and financial wealth. *Spending as consumption* uses up resources and squanders them.

Kiyosaki (1997):
> "When you work for money, *money controls your emotions*. Rich dad thought it foolish to spend your life working for money and to pretend that money was not important. He believed that life was more important than money, but money was important for supporting life."

Setting Money Limits

If you need to set limits on money, on your meanings about what money is and what it can do, what are some of those limits? And how do you set the limits on money?

The first limit is the limit on what money can and cannot buy. Do you know that? How well do you know that? Look at your list of all the things you want from money (Figure 4:2). Can money buy any of these things? That's a rhetorical question. Of course it cannot! Yet how well do you know that? How deep is that knowledge inside you? Is that deep enough for you to avoid becoming addicted to meaning?

What can money buy? Make a list of the things that you do want that money *can buy*. Now make a list of the things you always wanted money for that money *cannot buy*. The fact is that money cannot *buy* happiness, peace of mind, security, satisfaction, appreciation, health, etc. Money cannot even solve poverty.

Isn't that last statement a shocking realization? Money cannot even solve poverty! That's because merely giving people money does not make them wealthy. Even a million dollars would not make them wealthy. That's because *if* they do not know how to create wealth with their money, it is just a matter of time and they will have nothing left. And this happens to be the story of so many lottery winners. Being poor inside, being poverty-minded, lacking the wealth-creating capacity, the windfall of money simply came in and went out.

They were given a fish, and for awhile, they had plenty. But they never learned to fish. So after the consumption of the money, they were back to where they started, no richer and actually considerably poorer for the experience.

Perhaps that explains what Ted Turner said to Barbara Walters. Do you know what he said when she asked him, "How does it feel to be so rich?" As a billionaire, she wanted to know how it felt. He said:

"It's a paper sack. [pause] ... Everybody wants the paper sack. But when you reach in, it's just a handful of air."

By contrast, do you know what John D. Rockefeller said when he was asked, "How much more do you need?" He was asked this when he was a billionaire. And his answer is as telling as it is sad. He said, "Just one dollar more." Imagine that. He didn't have enough! Apparently he had not put a limit on money and so was desperate for more.

It is this addictive nature of money that shouts at us to set a limit for our need for money. When will you have enough? When will you say, "Enough!"? When will you check off: "Wealthy enough"? There is something addictive about success, achievement, power, and money which suggests that you need to beware lest you build the frame, "Just a little more." That actually is the definition of greed. And greed is a state that keeps you never able to relax and enjoy the abundance. No wonder it is not a very pleasant or desirable state. It damages you as it induces a state of discontent.

- How can you keep your ambitions *and* at the same time relax and enjoy life in the process?
- How can you feel satisfaction and yet stay ambitious about your goals?
- How much money is enough money?

The fact that wealth itself typically enlarges your appetite for riches, rather than satisfies it, is what makes wealth itself dangerous. The majority of success-driven people believe and operate from the perspective that "Enough is never enough." They always want 10% more, 25% more, 100% more, etc. If the drive to acquire more is not calmed with acquisition, what can calm it? We can calm it by setting limits and by shifting our focus to emphasize *being* more than *getting*.

What then is the best way to define money and what it can do? *It is just money*—it is a means of exchange, a way to measure what a culture values, what people will pay for. It is a scorecard and a resource, and that's all. It is not the purpose of life. And you will not take a dime of it with you!

My Personal Story
When I began wealth creation, I had a lot of negative and conflictive meanings about money and wealth. I had tried to set down several times

to write a wealth creation plan without success. Each time I started to do that, I would interrupt and distract myself. In fact, it was so subtle that I didn't even noticed. Eventually I did become aware of the unpleasantness and "struggle" involved in writing a plan. Once that awareness broke through I began to take notice. That's when I did the sentence-completion exercise.

"What wealth means to me..."
"To become wealthy I'd have to..."

It was the second one sentence-stem that really opened things up so that I could identify the things "in the back of the mind" which were holding me back. "To become wealthy I'd have to..."

"... refocus everything on money and become money-focused."
"... work really hard at things I don't enjoy."
"... take advantage of people."
"... become secular and materialistic."

When I began to free-flow allowing whatever was in the back of my mind to express itself, these were the kinds of things that came out. And I remember thinking about these things the question arose, "Where is all of this coming from?" When I got them down on paper, I sat back and thought, "You know, I don't even believe these things. So how is it that they are there, in my mind, holding me back?"

I then realized that many of them came from my dad and from some of the things he said as I was growing up. "Money doesn't grow on trees." "Wealthy people are greedy and stingy and get their money by taking advantage of others." Well, he grew up during the Great Depression. He was five years old in 1929 when the Stock Market crashed and so through his most formative years, there was not enough; there weren't enough jobs; banks were failing; and so he joined the army at 19 for World War II for two reasons, one of which was to have a job. No wonder he believed these things, which by the 1960s were no longer true and certainly not true for the cultural environment in which I lived.

Identifying these limiting and sabotaging ideas as some of the meanings governing my unconscious thinking and feeling about money and wealth enabled me to then do something about them. I changed them. I quality controlled them to determine which supported me and which limited me. Then I reframed them for more enhancing meanings about money.

The Main Points of this Chapter
The meanings that you give to wealth, money, and all of the facets involved in creating wealth *play a central and critical role.* If you give these two ideas (money and wealth) the wrong meanings—inadequate meanings, distorted meanings, pathological meanings—you will undermine your ability to create wealth and distort the experience itself. Conversely, building your understanding about wealth, and wealth creation, with rich and robust meanings enables the process.

As a meaning-maker, the kind and quality of meanings that you give to these things can accurately map out the process or over-load it semantically making you liable for money addiction. To think like a millionaire begins here. There is more, much more, and we will cover those steps in the next chapter.

Your Adventure in Creating Wealth
Coaching time! Are you ready to continue your wealth adventure? If so, then as your wealth coach, get your Wealth Adventure Journal and write out your sentence completions to these sentence stems:
> *"I know I will be wealthy when ..."*
> *"True wealth for me is..."*
> *"The wealth that I want and will pursue is .."*

Once you complete that, you are ready to write your first definition of "wealth"—the definition that you want to govern the direction of your wealth creation activities. Remember, it is better to start with some definition of wealth and refine and hone it over time than to put it off waiting until you have a definition that gives you an Eureka Experience!

After you complete the checklist with Figure 4:2, identify the links and associations you have made to wealth that over-loads it. What will you begin doing this week to unload that much meaning from your wealth associations?

End of Chapter Notes
1: See *Games Fit and Slim People Play* (2001) for a description of psycho-eating. This refers to emotional eating—eating for psychological reasons other than nutrition, metabolism, energy, and vitality. It is eating for love, reward, affection, power, de-stressing, the good life, and other psychological reasons—hence, psycho-eating.

Chapter 5

WHAT ARE THE BEST MEANINGS FOR WEALTH CREATION?

"The man who does not work for the love of work, but only for the money is not likely to make money, nor to find much fun in life."
Charles M. Schwab

"Faith makes thoughts real, it's the chemist of the mind."
How? By repeating affirmation.
It translates thoughts into physical equivalent
and creates a state of expecting.
Those who succeed develop
a passion for changing their minds,
from a failure consciousness to a success consciousness."
Napoleon Hill (p. 28, 50)

Meaning plays an incredibly powerful and subtle influence on your ability to create wealth. I hope that realization was one of the *Ahas!* from the previous chapter. What you think it is, and how to create it, constitutes your mental map for navigating the territory of wealth creation. In the previous chapter you were invited to identify and expand your meanings about wealth and about money. The richness and quality of the meanings you give to wealth and wealth creation determine how meaningful it will be to you. And that will empower your intention and long-term motivation. In this chapter we continue our exploration into meaning as we identify the very heart of wealth—what it is, some of the forms that meaning can take, and how to actualize your wealth potentials.

The Heart of Wealth
Having developed a healthy wealth orientation and a prosperity attitude is not enough to be ready to create wealth. More is needed. You need something else, you need to know *the essence* of wealth—*how* wealth is created and what *you* can do to create it. When you know the heart of wealth, you can go into a very special state of mind-and-emotion. So here's a test: Do you know what that is?

Let's begin by making a list of words that all seem to refer to this domain. Doing that gives us a list like this: wealth, money, value, valuing, appreciate, rich, enrich, worth, appraisal, prosperity, abundance, resources, affluence, etc.

Wealth obviously relates to what is valued. If you have plenty of what you and others do not value, is that wealth? If it is valued, appreciated, and highly esteemed, then it must be seen as offering a resource that gives worth and value to your life or the lives of others. What is valued? We value what makes our lives easier, more effective, more efficient, and more fun. We value things that gratify our basic and higher needs—survival, safety, love and affection, self-value and dignity, self-actualization. We value and buy what we think or what our culture tells us is important to the quality, improvement, and enrichment of our life and our relationship.

This explains why wealth changes from culture to culture and from age to age. Once wealth meant having a castle, soldiers, horses, swords, knights, etc. Once wealth meant having a scribe to write edicts and letters for you. Now anyone with a computer and a junior high school education is richer than Kings and majestrates in former ages.

> **The *essence* of wealth is using your talents, passions, and circumstances to *value, add value, and create things and experiences that people value.***

If wealth is value, how is wealth created? Wealth is created by creating ideas, experiences, and products that people want and value. Wealth is created by anything that adds value to people's lives. All of this means that *wealth* itself (as a concept rather than a thing) is fluid and flexible depending on what you and others say is valuable. That's why the process of creating wealth involves finding and inventing valuable things and/or making what people already have more valuable.

Wealth is relative to whatever we humans value, find valuable, or think gives value. That's why in every culture there are different standards and criteria for wealth, and why it keeps changing. The bottom line?

> *The heart of wealth is creating* or *adding value that meets the needs of people in a given context. Do that and the money will follow.*

For your own inside-out wealth the first application should be to yourself—*add value to your mind, emotions, skills, interests, passions, and relationships.* Become richer and more resourceful within yourself. This is *being*-wealth and *being*-wealth comes first. It comes a long time before the *doing* wealth that gives value to others. It also comes before the *having* wealth of owning the possessions and luxury items that you want.

No wonder wealth is not money. Money is a symptom of wealth, but not its core. Money only measures how you count the value of a given thing, product, service, or information. And that reason

> Wealth is value; it is what is valued. It is valued products and services that add to the quality of life.

explains why these things and experiences can gain or lose value (=wealth). This also explains how supply-and-demand come into the picture adding another complicating variable. One irony is that the more successful you are at creating a valuable product for a market, the more others will enter into that field to supply that need or want, the more likely that will then bring the price down.

Your personal wealth is whatever you value. Wealth for others is whatever they value. No wonder *wealth* and *value* are synonyms. Yet linguistically both of these words are nominalizations, that is, they are verbs-turned-into-nouns. So while "wealth" and "value" sound like things, they are not. The actual

> **Principle:**
> Your personal wealth is created through finding a passion and giving yourself to it for a decade or more as you develop your expertise is creating and giving value.

process is *creating* wealth or *creating value* or *valuing*. How is this linguistic analysis important? It enables you to see that the essence of wealth is creating ideas, products, services, relationships, etc. which you and others consider significant and important.

And Now— the State

If wealth is value, what then is *the state* and *the experience* when you experience wealth? How do you experience wealth as a state?

Get ready for an Aha! *The experience and state of wealth is the experience of appreciating.* You appreciate a solution to a need—a value for a context. The experience is *feeling rich* —abundant, full, resourceful in handling the requirements of life. The experience is *esteeming* and appraising the importance, value, significance, and meaningfulness of what you can do to increase the value of something.

Ah, another *Aha* moment! Or did you miss it? If so, go back and reread the previous paragraph. Then take a few moments to reflect on what it means, or could mean, for you. When I first did, I began to realize that *it is the state of appreciation that makes me rich.* In other words, I become richer every time I appreciate even if I am only appreciating one of the smallest things of life.

So to begin to experience this, take an inventory of all the things you value and appreciate about yourself, your life, others. Your ability to appreciate increases your sense of wealth. Inner wealth describes an affluence of your spirit to see the value of things and where you do that the meaningfulness of life expands.

Wealth involves the three dimensions of experience in this order: being—doing —having. The *being* states of wealth come first and comprises the core. And at the core is valuing— appreciating. This leads to your sense of self-wealth in your sense of self-esteem and self-efficacy. Who you *are* as a person is valuable and knowing that frees you to learn and develop certain things that you can *do* that adds value to others. That gives you the *doing* wealth states and that leads to the *having* wealth states. And within the doing and having is the heart-pulse of appreciation.

> "Always pretend that you're working for yourself. You'll do a wonderful job in that case. If you are finding that you don't love your job or that you're not doing a good job, demand a meeting with your boss immediately. If the situation doesn't improve, fire yourself (and your boss) and go do something else." Donald Trump (81)

What is your personal process for creating wealth?
Because as all of this opens up the essence of wealth, and therefore of wealth creation, it enables you to find your way to create wealth. How will you create wealth?

You create wealth best by using your valuable *being* and *doing* states for the purpose of adding value to others. As you value and appreciate what you add that makes a difference, and care about doing so, you are then able to become completely absorbed in it. You become passionately committed to it. And you delightfully thrill in developing your skills and expertise in creating it for others.

This is the point Napoleon Hill drove home in all his books, namely, that all achievement and all earned riches, have their beginning in *an idea*—the passionate idea of how you can add value. He also said that desire was the starting point for all achievement, and so he encouraged people to cultivate a white hot desire so that it becomes a keen, pulsating force.

Stanley (2000) in *The Millionaire Mind* described this pulsating force using a different terminology— the language of love:
> "If you *love what you are doing,* your productivity will be high and your specific form of creative genius will emerge." (p. 61)

> Martha Sinetar:
> "The task is easier than people imagine. All it takes is everything they have to give: all their talent, energy, focus, commitment and all their love." (p. 7)

This has been known for a long time. At the turn of the twentieth century Booker T. Washington (1901) wrote to African Americans, long before civil rights, spoke about the heart of wealth creation as *adding value*. And he should know— his genius and creativity in solving technical problems and adding value was the heart of his own success.
> "When a girl learns to cook, to wash dishes, to sew, to write a book, or a boy learns to groom horses, or to grow sweet potatoes, or to produce butter, or to build a house, or to be able to practice medicine, as well or better than someone else, they will be rewarded regardless of race or color. In the long run, the world is going to have the best, and any difference in race, religion, or previous history will not long keep the world from its wants.

"I think that the whole future of my race hinges on the question of whether or not it can make itself of such indispensable value that the people in the town and the state where we reside will feel that our presence is necessary to the happiness and well-being of the community.
No man who continues to add something to the material, intellectual, and moral well-being of the place in which he lives is long left without proper reward. This is a great human law which cannot be permanently nullified." (p. 149)

Now that you have in your mental possession the secret regarding the essential core of wealth creation, what will you do with this secret? How will you use this to unleash your wealth potentials?

> *It is the state of appreciation that makes me rich.*

Figure 5:1
Actualizing Your Wealth Potentials

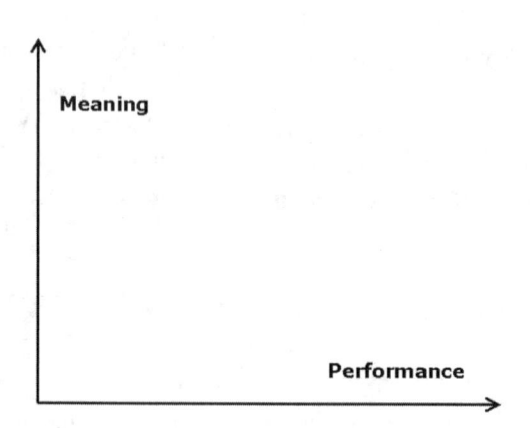

[Graph with vertical axis labeled "Meaning" and horizontal axis labeled "Performance"]

What does it take to actualize or make real your potentials for creating wealth? It takes the same two things that it takes to actualize any and all of your potentials. That's because self-actualization is a function of two key factors. I discovered and wrote about these two factors of self-actualization in *Unleashed* (2007) and in *Self-Actualization Psychology*

(2008). What are these two factors?
> *Actualizing your highest and best potentials is a function of meaning and performance.*

To actualize anything, you have to see it as *meaningful* (significant, important, and valuable) and you have to take actions to give those meanings a real-world *performance.* When human beings have actualized their highest and best, they have met these two criteria. First, it *meant* a lot to them. Usually it meant the world to them. They were passionate about it and made it their first, and sometimes only, priority. Then second, it was something that the person *acted on* and *lived for.*

In Neuro-Semantics the combination of meaning and performance has led to the development of the Self-Actualization Quadrants. Using *meaning* and *performance* as the vertical and horizontal axes gives us four possible spaces where you can be in actualizing anything, including your wealth potentials.

> "From my career of studying wealthy people and an interview with sixty millionaires I learned that ... You cannot enjoy life if you are addicted to consumption and the use of credit."
> Thomas Stanley
> *The Millionaire Mind*

You can now use these two axes and four quadrants to identify where you are in terms of your development.

I: Low meanings and low performance means no motivation, no vision, no dreams, and no actions. This is where we all start and where we are when we are undeveloped in terms of our meanings and performances. It is also here that we fall back to when disillusioned.

II: High meanings with low performance means unfulfilled dreams. When we are here, we have developed only our mind to dream about possibilities and to create the inspiration about what we would like to do.

III: High performance with low meanings. This is on the performance scale. With high performance and low meanings you are able to do a lot, achieve a lot, and perhaps even make a lot of money which enables you to reach high levels of success, status, recognition, but it will mean very little. Somehow it doesn't count, it is not significant or meaningful —perhaps it comes too easy. If you then keep working hard doing more, you are likely to burn-out.

IV: High meanings and high performance is the ideal quadrant since it is here that you fulfill your dreams and make real your visions. Here meaning and performance synergize.

Figure 5:2

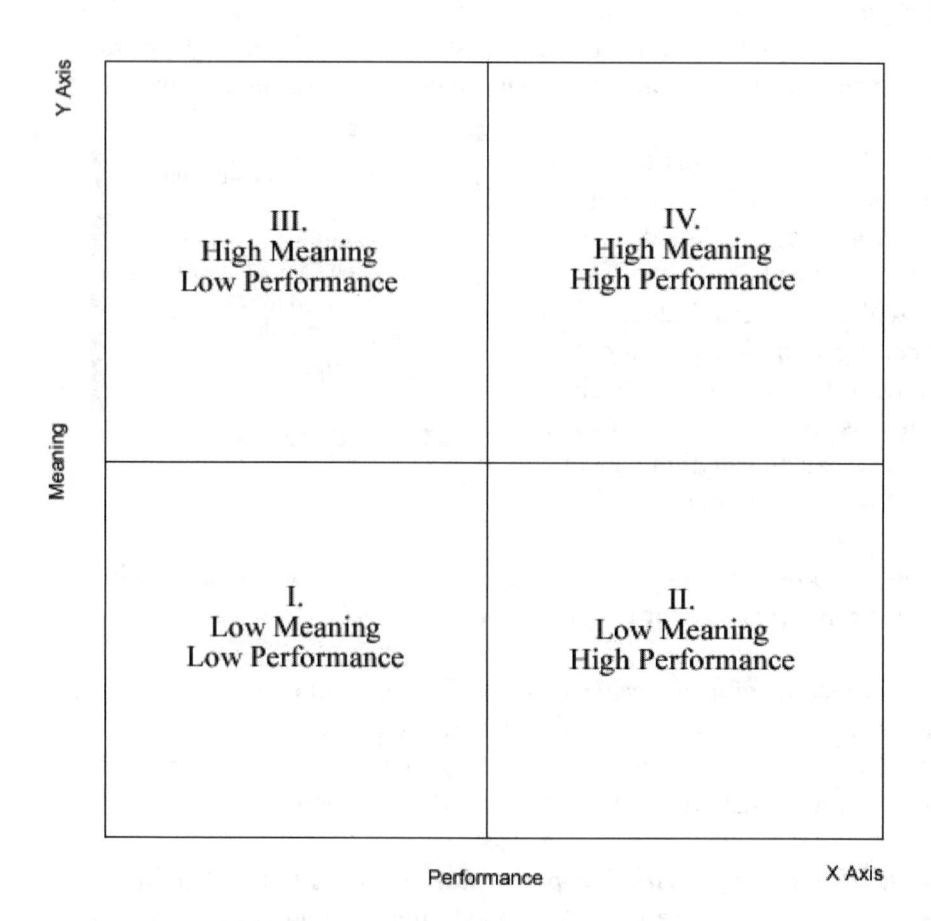

III. High Meaning Low Performance	IV. High Meaning High Performance
I. Low Meaning Low Performance	II. Low Meaning High Performance

Y Axis — Meaning
X Axis — Performance

Let's label the four quadrants. Quadrant I is the *Undeveloped Quadrant* and includes "the pit of disillusionment" for people in Quadrants II and III when they overdo their strength and discover that it does not lead them to the self-actualization quadrant. Quadrant II is *Performers;* Quadrant III is *Dreamers*. That leaves Quadrant IV, *Self-Actualizers*. Quadrant IV is where you make things happen by synergizing meaning and performance.

So how do you actualize your wealth potentials? *You synergize your meanings* (and your highest meanings) *with your best performances.* You combine into an optimal response your values and your actions. You act on what inspires you and the activities that you do as part of your wealth creation plan, you endow with rich meanings. So which is your natural tendency? What do you tend to default to when things don't go as they should? Which axis (meaning or performance) will you need to develop?

Forms of Meaning
All this talk about meaning typically invites the questions:
> "What is meaning anyway? What do you mean by meaning? Are you talking about beliefs or understanding or concepts or what?"

Short and quick, *meaning is anything and everything you hold in mind.* That's the literal definition of the term, "to hold in mind." So whatever you keep in mind, hold in your thinking and emoting, that is your meaning. And there are many, many forms of meaning, that is, many ways for meaning to be coded. What are these codes? Among the most common are the following:

Representations
Attentions
Perceptions
Beliefs
Understandings
Concepts
Metaphors
Words, language, phrases
Evaluations
Permissions or prohibitions
Decisions, choices

> **Psycho-logical:** We are not a logical species, but *psycho*-logical. Our logics are based on the references that we apply to our thinking, feeling, and experiencing.

Your meanings and mine most commonly take the form of beliefs, decisions, and representations. As we start there, it leads to what we call meta-questions—questions about the structure and form of "thinking."[1]
• What are you representing in your mind?
• What do you believe about that?
• What thoughts or images come to mind?
• What have you decided about that? Is that your choice?
• What do you understand about that?

These categories give us a way to flush out meanings. And that is because your meanings are mostly unconscious. As meaning frames—you live *inside* them to such an extent that you don't notice the frame itself. Like Neo in the Matrix, the Matrix *has* you. Your matrix of beliefs, decisions, understandings, memories, imaginations, etc. *have* you. And it will continue to have you until you become aware of it. Then you can develop the ability to step in and out of that Matrix at will. When you develop that skill, then you become the one —the master of your matrix of meanings.[2]

Figure 5:3
The Power of Meanings as Beliefs

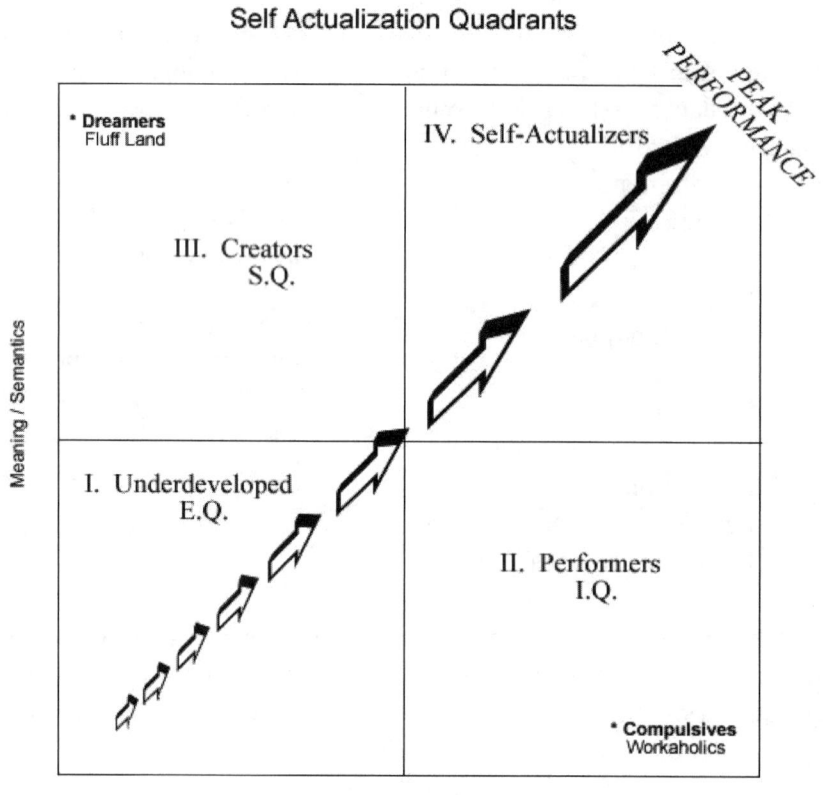

Self Actuialization Quadrants

- **Dreamers**
  Fluff Land

III. Creators
S.Q.

IV. Self-Actualizers

PEAK PERFORMANCE

I. Underdeveloped
E.Q.

II. Performers
I.Q.

- **Compulsives**
  Workaholics

Meaning / Semantics

Performance / Neuro-Physiology

When you encode your meanings as beliefs, you create a very powerful psychological mechanism. That's because beliefs operate as self-fulfilling prophecies and organize you psycho-logically. They create your psycho-logical fate. That is, once you set a belief, that belief sets your fate—your direction and orientation. And as a "belief" you will tend to uncritically accept it without question. And as you live within it, it operates as your world— your Matrix world. This means that as you take your beliefs for granted, your beliefs define your "sense of reality"—what's real, what's possible, what you can do, what you deserve, what to focus on, what things mean, what causes things, etc. "As you believe—so you are."[3]

What fate "logically" has to occur in your life because of your beliefs about money, wealth, or some aspect of your finances? Do these consequences serve you well? Would you like to change them? How much would you like to transform them?

> "I can never stand still. I must explore and experiment. I am never satisfied with my work. I resent the limitations of my own imagination." ... "Money—or rather the lack of it to carry out my ideas—may worry me, but it does not excite me. Ideas excite me." ... "The Dreamer focuses on the 'big picture' with the attitude that anything is possible."
> (Dilts about the Disney genius) *Disney Animation: The Illusion of Life*, by F. Thomas and O. Johnson (1981, p. 25, 168, 185)

Here's something else powerful and frightening about beliefs —*beliefs operate as commands to your nervous system.* Thoughts send signals or messages to the body, but beliefs do much more. They send *commands* for responses from your entire neurology and all of your nervous systems. This explains the power of a belief to effect you so powerfully. So, what commands have you given to your nervous system, brain, neurology, etc.?

Now if you are ready for something really crazy, consider this. *Your belief does not have to be "true" to be believed.* We all have believed lots of things that turned out to not be true, haven't we? Haven't you? You and I can *feel* that a belief is real and true, and be fully convinced of it, and later find out that our belief was actually based on false information. Richard Bandler speaks about this:

> "It doesn't matter if it's true or not — it only matters that you have the belief, that you will do it with every fiber of your muscles and your soul." (Bandler, 1985, p. 80)

Anti-Wealth Building Beliefs:
Do you have any beliefs about wealth, about wealth creation, about saving, spending, budgeting, etc. that hold you back? What meaning do you have as a belief that might operate as a limiting belief within you? In the following examples, check those that you believe or that you may think that you believe at an unconscious level:

> To make a lot of money takes a lot of hard work.
> Making money is highly stressful.
> I'll never have enough.
> I can't learn all of this! It's too overwhelming.
> I don't know if I deserve to be wealthy.
> What about all the starving people in the world?
> What if I become a selfish snot when I get rich?
> Money is evil.
> Money doesn't grow on trees.
> Rich people screw the poor.
> You'd have to sell drugs to make lots of money.

What are some empowering beliefs about wealth and wealth creation? What could you believe that would help to establish a mind-set that supports wealth and wealth creation? Here is a list of beliefs that you could possibly install to assist you. Check those that you would like to believe— that if you did believe, that belief would make a positive difference for you:

> I can identify my talents and do what I set my mind to do.
> I have a big *why* for creating a fortune.
> I can confidently take insightful action to make my goals real.
> Money is a resource not to be squandered.
> I can develop clear and specific goals.
> I can enjoy working and turning the work into play.
> I can work hard for what I believe in.
> I can love what I do and view it as a privilege.
> I can take charge of my own destiny.
> Every problem has dozens of good solutions.
> There are always solutions.
> It never hurts to ask for what I want.
> Nearly everything is negotiable.
> Risk isn't working for yourself, risk is working for someone else.
> I can and will solve problems.
> Solving problems is fun.
> I will become a CEO by owning my own company.

There are no limits on the amount of income I can make.
I get stronger and wiser every day by facing risk and adversity.
No matter what comes along, I can figure out a solution; there's always a solution.
Paying my dues is just part of the process.
If I don't risk anything, I will never gain anything. Risking is the way to greatness.
Becoming more and more resourceful is a learnable skill.
More is not necessarily better— higher quality, more alignment with values and visions is better.
Commitment is the key to excellence.
The more I extend myself to others, the more people I'll influence for good.
I, along with every human being, deserve to succeed.
I can play at the work as my strategy for success.
Life is more important than money and that money is important for supporting life.
I can and will walk away from every negotiation that isn't a Win/Win deal.
I can find many new ways to add value to what I do.

As you meditate on this list, create your own personalized list of empowering beliefs that will beef up your attitude about work, saving, budgeting, investing, studying, selling, finding your niche, etc. As you do this, avoid asking if you believe it, only focus on this:

> Would you like to believe it? Would that belief be ecological, empowering for you, and useful?

A final thing about beliefs; they can be well-formed or ill-formed. If you want your beliefs to be well-formed beliefs, then formulate the beliefs using the following distinctions. I have used one of my beliefs as an example:

Well-Formed Belief Criteria
1) State the belief in the affirmative.
> "I believe wealth is created by adding value to people in the things I do."

2) State it an as action that you can do. Make it actionable.
> "I believe I can add value by the problems I can solve that enriches the lives of people."

3) State it as a map about your direction and the processes you will use.

Does your statement give direction, create perspective, facilitate a decision for you?

> "I believe I can find and develop my ability to add value in the books I write by giving explicit instructions on how to do things."

4) State it as an operationalized set of actions.

> "Because I believe I can use my study and research skills to expand my ability to find new creative solutions so people can unleash their financial potentials, I will keep refining my training materials and books, testing them with real live people, look for how to make it more practical, understandable, and actionable."

5) State something that is meaningful and compelling to you.

> "I believe that as I learn more and experience more in wealth creation, I can unleash the wealth creation in thousands of others, and turn loose thousands of people, who will make the lives of millions richer."

Meta-Yes-ing for Transforming Thoughts into Beliefs

Once you have discovered some limiting beliefs that you want to get out of your head and neurology so that they no longer operate as your programming, you can use the Meta-State pattern that we call *Meta-Yes-ing* for changing limiting beliefs.[4] This process will give you a clear, quick, and effective way to deframe the old unenhancing beliefs and to install the empowering beliefs that support your commitment to success.

To prepare for this pattern you first have to decide upon the limiting belief to change and the new empowering belief to replace it with. There is no "ecology" inside of the pattern, only at the beginning and then afterwards as you step back to evaluate the end result. So here are a set of questions for deciding on what beliefs to change and which to install:

- What enhancing and empowering beliefs would you really like to have running in your mind-and-emotions?
- Which belief stands in your way from wealth building?
- How does this belief sabotage you or undermine your effectiveness?
- Have you had enough of it? Or do you need more pain?
- What empowering belief would you like to have in its place?

Once you have identified a limiting belief that gets in your way and sabotages your wealth creation, access a state where you feel a strong sense of refusal, of *"No!"* Now to do this you will need to think about something very negative that every fiber in your body would never allow you to experience. So begin to think of something that every fiber in your body says *"No!"* to in a fully congruent way. Examples that I like using with people are these: Would you push a little child in front of a speeding bus just for the hell of it? Would you eat a bowl of dirty filthy worms when you have delicious food available?

How strong of a "No!" response do these questions elicit in you? If there is an absolute sense of "No!" inside, then say that "No!" repeatedly and notice the qualities that you bring to it—the volume of your voice, your tone, your firmness, etc. Notice how it feels. Notice your body posture, your gestures, etc. Now anchor your "No!" with your hand gestures. How do you say "No" with your hands? I do so by pushing my hands away from my body straight in front of me, with my palms facing upward. Feel the negation as you gesture it.

When you have a strong sense of "No!" say it to the limiting belief that gets in your way. Imagine that belief is out in front of you and someone offering it to you. Do you want it? Does it serve you? Enhance your life? As you consider these questions and respond with a "No," keep saying it until you access a very strong and powerful *"No!"* If appropriate, turn it up to a sense of, *"Hell No!"* Now feel this fully as you think about that stupid, useless, limiting belief.

How long should you keep saying *No!* to that limiting belief? Do it until you feel that it no longer has any power to run your programs, that it has no more room in your presence, in your mind. Now ask this question of yourself: How many more times, and with what voice, tone, gesturing, do you need to totally disconfirm that old belief so that you know —deep inside yourself—that it will no longer run your thinking and acting?

Once you've done that, literally and physically move away from where you expressed the *No,* and access a strong and robust *"Yes!"* To do that, think about something—anything—that every fiber of your being can say *"Yes!"* to without any question or doubt. Do you have something like that? Again, notice your *"Yes!"* Notice the neurology and feeling of your *"Yes!"* Notice the voice of "Yes!" Gesture the "Yes!" with your hands and body. Amplify this "Yes!" By way of contrast, I hold my hands– palm up— with fingers moving forward to me as if to say, "come here, come to me. You are welcomed."

When you feel that you have a fantastic *:Yes* state, then take that *"Yes!"* and apply it to your new enhancing belief. Doing this is meta-stating the thought so that it becomes a belief. Pose questions to yourself that imply a *yes* answer.

> Do you want this? Would it make things better? Would it enable you to move forward in creating the wealth that you want?

The design here is to bring that *yes* and the feeling of that *"Yes!"* to the empowering belief and to do so repeatedly. Do you want this? *"Yes!"* Really? Finally, ask yourself this question:

> How many more times do you need to say "Yes!" right now in order to feel that you have fully welcomed it into your presence?

The next step will seem a little strange at first. Now say *"Yes"* to the *"Yes!"* which you said to the new belief and do this repeatedly. To do this, pose such questions to yourself as the following:

> So do you think that this belief is something that you really want? Would you like to keep that new belief? Are you going to?

In *meta-yes-ing* you are expressing a state of validation to a thought. It is the validation state that transforms a thought into something more, into a belief. Keep repeating this process until when you think of the new thought, you have an immediate response within yourself that goes, "Of Course."

My Personal Story
When I compare my beliefs now to those I had about money, wealth, wealth creation, etc., my first beliefs were small, minimal, and very cautious. "I believe I can double my income in five years." That was a hard one. At the time I was making $25,000 a year (in a good year), and the idea that I could make $50K income was outrageous, incredible, and preposterous. "Would I *like* to believe it?" Sure! But really, let's be realistic! How could I ever make $50K in a single year?! I didn't realize it at the time, but the problem wasn't the numbers, the problem was my limiting beliefs. I was undermining myself by using my current experiences and reality to question that desired belief.

Three years later when my income reached $50K, I added a new belief. "I believe I can make $100K a year." And again, that seemed preposterous. In fact, I remember thinking as I first thought, "Well, not really. That's just not realistic." A few years later, having made that amount for several years in a row, I really went wild. "I believe it is possible for me to make one million dollars a year in income." [As of this writing I have not yet made a million dollars in a year, but I now truly believe that I can, that it is a realistic possibility.]

"I believe I can create a business—several businesses." Beliefs are powerful mental maps about what's possible, what things mean, who we are, what causes the effects that we want, what is important, etc. And the wondrous thing about beliefs is that we — you and I— are not stuck with our beliefs. We can change them. We can update them. We can clean them up. We can eradicate impurities and distortions within them.

Your Adventure in Creating Wealth
As your Wealth Coach, your task this week is to make a list each day of *ten things you appreciate today.* The things you appreciate may be the same things each day or different things. After a week of making appreciation lists, create a full list of all the things you appreciate.
> How easy or difficult is this for you? As you reflect on your ability to appreciate, what criteria do you use to decide on what to appreciate?

Next, take your ability to appreciation and apply to yourself as a wealth creator. What values are you able to deliver to others?

Here's your next assignment: Explore your beliefs about wealth. What do you believe about wealth? About money? Make a list of beliefs that you have about these subjects. Find someone to talk about creating wealth and notice the things you say. When you identify some limiting beliefs, formulate what you would prefer to believe that would be positive and empowering for you. Now run the Meta-Yes-ing pattern on those beliefs.

End of Chapter Notes

1: Meta-Questions refer to higher level questions, questions not about the outside external world (when, where, who, what, etc.), but about your internal world. These questions takes you *up* into a person's frames of mind to understand their meaning matrix and the inner world from which they operate. And that provides a place for transformational change.

2: The Matrix Model provides a way to distinguish eight key factors that create and reflect our reality. See *The Matrix Model* (2003) or the Neuro-Semantic training, *Matrix Training*.

3: The terminology of our psycho-logics comes from Alfred Korzybski (1933). For more about semantic loading and the psycho-logics of our lives see *Meta-States* (2005) or *Winning the Inner Game* (2007).

4: For more about the *Meta-Yes* structure, see *Sub-Modalities Going Meta* (2005). There are also numerous articles and patterns on the Meta-Yes Belief Change pattern on the website, www.neurosemantics.com.

PART II

THE CORE OF

WEALTH CREATION

The core of wealth creation is to identity the interface between your potential and passion with an economic context whether a product, service, experience, or business that adds tremendous value for people. This interface is *the Singularity*.

Chapter 6

HOW DO I GET STARTED?

*"If you expect your money to take care of you,
you must take care of your money."*
Suze Orman (1999)

*"There are as many CEOs living paycheck to paycheck
as there are secretaries."*
Machtig and Behrends (p. 35)

Let's say that you have decided to create wealth and to become a wealth creator. Let's say that you have a vision and dream of how to create wealth through a product, service, experience, or business. Let's say that you feel passionate about this, have high level intentions for doing this, and have made an informed decision to make this happen.

- Now what? How do you get started?
- What's the first thing you do?

The answer, of course, is that it depends on where you are in the stages of wealth creation. Are you at the beginning, in the middle, or towards the end? Here I will describe the entire process. I will begin at the beginning and move through the stages of wealth creation. Because this chapter will enable you to identify where you are, you can use the stages as a checklist for the steps you have already achieved, and those yet to come.

Economics 101
We begin with *Economics 101* to understand where money comes from, how it works, and what it takes to make lots of money. If creating financial wealth means making money, then how do we make money?

While that question sounds like the most simple and obvious question, it really is not. On the surface, you would think:
> "Sure, I know where money comes from; it comes from an employer paying your salary."

And yes, that's where the majority of people get their money. Yet that answer is actually not only inadequate, it is wrong. So let's ask yet another question, "Where does the employer get money to pay employees?" Ah, now we are getting closer.
> "Customers and clients pay employers for their products and services, that's where the money comes from."

Closer, and yet we still have not quite arrived at the source of where money comes from. Let's ask yet another question, "Why do customers and clients invest money into various products, services, and experiences? Why do they do that?" This question now brings us to the heart of things.
> *People buy things and experiences because they add value to their lives.*

You buy things to satisfy a need or a desire. You buy things to enrich your life. As human beings we spend money to make things better—solve problems, fulfil dreams, gratify the basic human needs, and/or delight in their highest self-actualization needs.

Money comes from adding value to people. The more value that a product, service, or experience adds—the more people value a particular product or service, the more money they will invest in that solution. So to make money, add value—add massive value, add life-enhancing value, and especially keep nurturing your golden goose—your value-adding capacity.

No business can continue to exist if it costs more to make and present its products and services than it charges. So first you need to be able to add value through the products and services you create and provide. This requires that you are able to find or create a market for the products and services, and that you create a business structure that enables you to generate a profit margin. Then if there is a demand for what you offer and you can supply that demand, you have the possibility of making money from it. This is Economics 101.

So how is money made?
> By creating value.
> By creating value for which there is a demand.
> By creating value that there will be a demand for when people find out about it.
> By creating a structure by which you can supply a solution for the demand whether a need or a desire.
> By letting people know what you offer, how it meets their needs, why it is important to them, and how they can obtain it.

If this is the heart of wealth creation, let's now ask the critical questions whereby you will be able to become a wealth creator. As these are questions for you to explore personally, I have put them in the first person:

- What value can I create and contribute?
- What skills and expertise do I have that can create desired value for people?
- What problems can I solve that people will pay to have solved?
- What dreams, hopes, and desires can I use my competencies to gratify?
- What will be involved in creating the product, service, or experience that will add value to people?
- Who will I need to be in order to become a part of the creation of this solution?
- What kind of a business structure will I need to find or build in order to deliver this value?
- How will I need to let people know the value that I can deliver?

These are the questions that you will need to answer to get started to make money and build the kind of financial wealth that you want. These questions also clarify why every wealth creation plan takes time. It takes time to identify the relationship between your skills and expertise, your interests and passions, the needs and desires of the market, and the business structure that will transfer the value.

So where do you start? All of the research convenes here—start with your current job. And if you don't have a job, get one. Any job. It doesn't matter. *What matters is your ability to add value in the context of serving customers.* And it doesn't matter if your customers are external or internal. What matters is how you treat them. The more you learn how to do these things, the more you will be able to create tremendous value (=money). That is absolutely critical. Can you do that? Will you do it? Since you have to start somewhere, and since the best place to start is where you are, then take *the wealth creation test.*

- Are you able to add value to customers and clients in your current job? To everyone who receives the result of your work?
- Are you able to use your skills and contribute something of value to those who receive your products or services?
- What is the value that you are adding?
- How can you add more value to what you are doing?
- How much better of an employee can you be?
- If you owned the business that you are working in, what would you do that would make it even better?

Answering these questions puts you well on your way to becoming a wealth creator. And do you know why that's so? Because you understand the heart and essence of wealth—*adding value.* And if you can't do it in your current job, or don't do it, the problem is either your belief, understanding, or your attitude.

"If I Owned this Place..."
I asked these questions and presented this approach once when I did the Wealth Creation training in Monterrey Mexico. At that training was a young man who had never kept a job for even a year. His problem? He was extremely impatient to get rich! He really wanted to be wealthy. There was no question about his motivation, he certainly had the desire. But he didn't have a marketable skill—he only had the passion. But something transformational happened to him in that three-day training.

An idea got into his mind. When I talked about going to work and adding value and looking at the business with the eyes of *"if I owned this place..."* something about that idea really appealed to him. He wanted to own it and so taking on that perception was a fabulous thought for him. And with that a transformation began. One that he didn't expect.

As he took that idea to work with him and operated from the frame of ownership, he began learning about business. He began thinking in terms of what do customers want? What can we offer? What are they getting now? From whom? How can we make a better offer? How can I add value to that customer? Within weeks, his employer started noticing him and at the end of that quarter he got his first raise—ever! At the end of the next quarter, he had earned another raise and so it went, quarter after quarter. And he began to realize what was happening—he was becoming a valuable employee, he was adding value to the company and to his employer.

That's when I got my first email from him. One year after the training, he wrote and said that someone from a competitor had come into the store, watched him, and then sent others to watch him. Eventually they hired him out of that company into another with a big increase in pay. A year after that he was made assistant manager, then manager. He kept me informed for several years and kept saying that it was all because of a single shift of perception—"If I owned this place what I would do is..."

The ownership perceptive essentially taught him the basics of Business 101 and enabled him to develop the heart of an entrepreneur. Paradoxically, it enabled him to get out of himself, and develop the ability to attend to the needs of others. And that tapped his capital of creativity and intelligence.

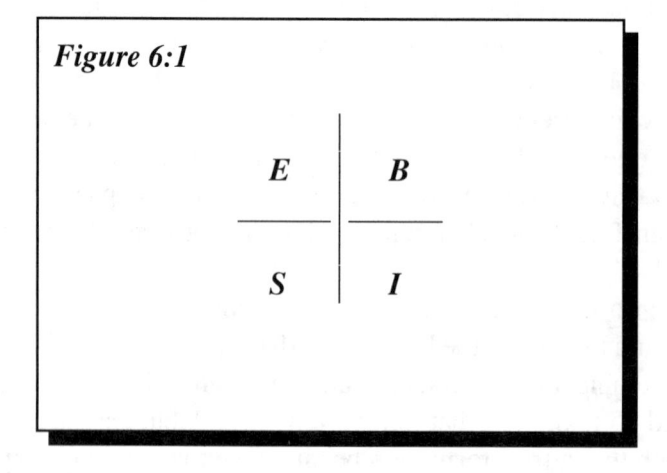

Figure 6:1

E	B
S	I

The Cashflow Quadrants

Robert Kiyosaki created the cashflow quadrants as a way to think about where money comes from and where you are in terms of either working for money or having money work for you. The cashflow quadrants simply identifies *the four sources of income:*

>   *E*mployee
>   *S*elf-Employee
>   *B*usiness Owner
>   *I*nvestor

Once while delivering the Wealth Creation Training in Avignon France, Denis Bridoux, a Neuro-Semantic NLP Trainer, who was doing the translating into French asked me about the quadrants. "What are the axes of the quadrants?" I had not given that any thought. So we engaged in a conversation to explore it. I tried to remember from my readings of Kiyosaki, but I wasn't sure. Eventually Denis and I came up with independence — interdependent and individual—group as possible or probable axes.

Using these distinctions led us to view the left side of the quadrants as the place where we all start. We work for someone as an employee or we work for ourselves as a self-employed employee. In both of these we work for money.

>   On the left side and at the top is *individual and dependence*—you are an individual Employee dependent on your employer for the job.
>   On the left side and at the bottom is *individual and independence*—you are an individual who is Self-Employed, now dependent on yourself to generate business and income.

It is in moving to the right side of the quadrants that things change and money works for us.

>   On the right side and at the bottom is the individual Investor who is a single individual.
>   On the right side and at the top is the Business owner who has a business.

When I got home a few weeks later, I found the book and so went back to the source. That's when I discovered that Kiyosaki had not built the quadrants around axes in the first place! He simply offered the four quadrants as four boxes or categories. The only structure for him was left side / right side. Left side—you work for money; right side—money works for you.

Figure 6:2

Left Side	Right Side
E	**B**
Employee We have a job We work for someone	**Business Owner** We own a system and people work for us. The business runs even when we are not there.
S	**I**
Self-Employed We own a job We work for ourselves	**Investor** Money works for us We invest our money

These four quadrants are simpler than what Denis and I had hallucinated. They simply identify *the different sources* of incomes. And Kiyosaki uses it to show that the most desirable choice is to move to, and operate from, the right side. That is, to become a business owner and/or an investor in businesses owned by others. If you want to build wealth aggressively, the sooner you move from working for others to working for yourself, the better. If you want to build wealth while maintaining your job and keeping the "security" of that income, then aim to build other sources of income outside your work hours.

To move from the employee and self-employed quadrants requires financial intelligence, a wealth creation plan, courage, and the willingness to invest in yourself. *Financial independence* arise from developing passive sources of income that exceed expenses. There are two ways to do that:

Figure 6:3
Re-Worked Diagram by Hall and Bridoux

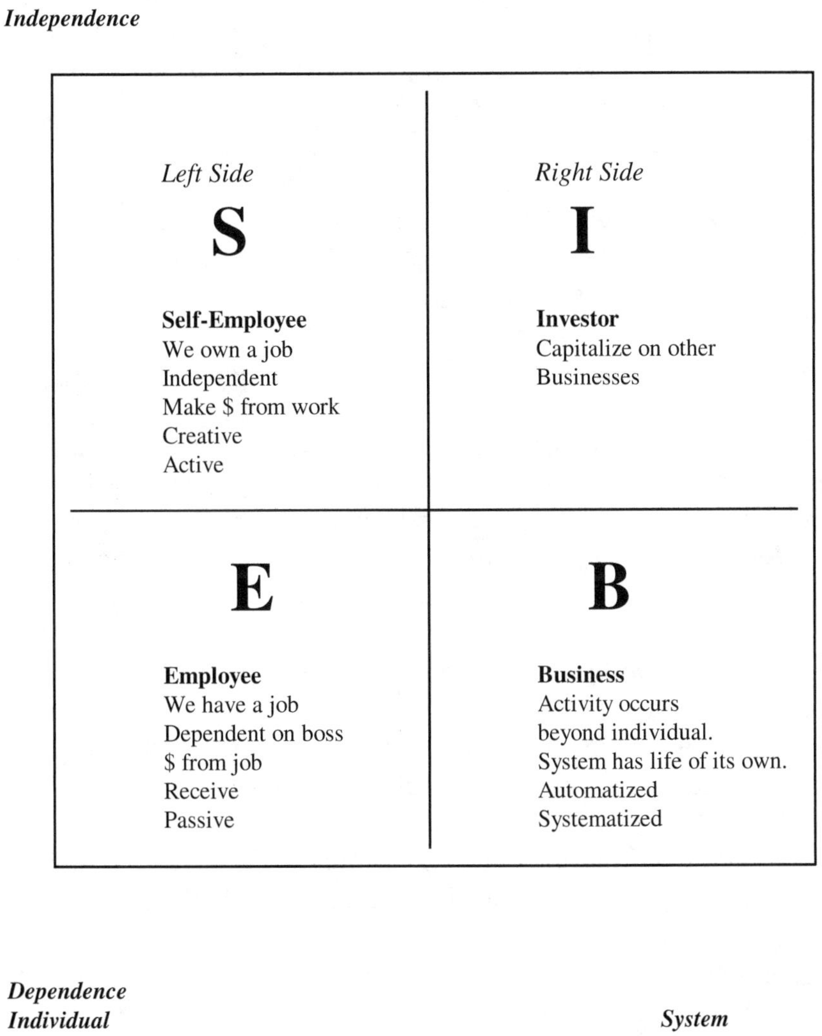

Independence

Left Side **S** **Self-Employee** We own a job Independent Make $ from work Creative Active	*Right Side* **I** **Investor** Capitalize on other Businesses
E **Employee** We have a job Dependent on boss $ from job Receive Passive	**B** **Business** Activity occurs beyond individual. System has life of its own. Automatized Systematized

Dependence
Individual   *System*

In Figure 6:3 Denis and I reorganized the quadrants using the X axis for dependence to independence and the Y axis for individual to system.

1) Develop and increase sources of passive income.
>Passive income means that once you've done the work, you don't have to keep putting in the same kind of energy ("word") to create the value. The system becomes self-sustaining or is sustained by a minimal amount of attention, effort, and time.

2) Reduce expenses.
>Develop efficiency in all of the processes that you use to create products and services. Quality control the processes to eliminate as much waste as possible. Open communication and participation as much as possible so employees become fully engaged in the process.

Initial Getting Started Steps
To make the getting started process explicit, let me summarize what to learn and do. Here are the first steps:

1) Realize how wealth arises and use that understanding to set your direction.
In a market driven economy, wealth is created by creating and selling products and services of value that individuals and groups want and will pay for. This generates money. To make money work for you, save and build up capital in order to create a process or company that intelligently uses these resources to generate ongoing business.

2) Practice value-adding by starting with your current job.
If you don't have a job, get one. If you have one, use it as your "Wealth Creation School." Study that business in order to understand fully how it works. Keep asking yourself business questions and wealth creation questions:
>What is the business strategy? What is the value that it is adding? How does it treat its customers—both the external and internal customers. How can you add value in your role? What are the numbers this business needs that make it work? What is the business model? How does it differ from others in this industry? What works really well? What doesn't work very well?

3) Develop and follow a budget.
Realizing that it's your job to create wealth and make yourself rich, and not your boss's job, or anyone else's, decide that you will take control

of your money. Begin that by creating a budget for your money. Your boss simply provides you a paycheck for the work you are contracted for. Your job is to make yourself financially viable, independent, and rich. This obviously requires self-discipline, awareness of income and expenses, willingness to budget, to not over-commit yourself to expenses and to wait until you have the money.

4) Get out of debt.
If you have debt, that debt is making someone other than you rich! So, *get rid of that kind of debt.* Treat indebtedness (i.e., school loans, loans on liabilities like car, boat, credit cards, etc.) as the sworn enemy to your financial stability and independence. Think of it as quicksand — devastating your financial foundations. Think of it as a thief of your capital and then go into battle against it. Eliminate all debt and only use debt, like that on a home, which truly benefits your long term investment. Spend less than you make or make more than you spend.

Credit card debts are among the worst kind of debts, especially if you are carrying balances over month to month. And this becomes doubly true if you are carrying debt on lifestyle items. That is a game that the financially-strapped play. And because it will undermine your wealth creation process, *stop it immediately.* Easy credit can seduce you into living high— living as if you're rich, yet the interest rate and the debt prevents you from becoming financially independent.

How can you defeat debt in your life? You will have to use all of the self-discipline, habits of frugality (squeezing all the joy out of the stuff that you do have), and commitment to your long term goals that you can muster.

> **The Budget Principle:**
> *Wealth is created by creating and following a budget to know where you are, what money is coming in, and where the money*

This preparation enables you to begin to think like a millionaire as you learn to resist being defeated in the game by impulsive spending, inability to resist immediate gratification, making long term plans, and developing the willingness to save and build capital.

And if you are deep in debt, how do you get out of that debt?
a) Make the commitment.
      The first wealth step is to make a commitment to get rid of your

debts. Every time you think about your debt, remind yourself that your debt is making someone else rich. If debt is consuming your time, energy, and creativity, you need first of all to aim to first reduce, and then eliminate, that debt.

b) Raise your debt awareness.

How much debt do you have? Do you even know how much debt you have? Track what you have coming in (income) and going out (expenses) so you can set a budget to keep expenses down.

c) Pay with cash.

Decide on a completely new and radical *modus operandi*. Decide that you will patiently save up for what you want, and buy only what you have cash to pay for. Are you willing to do that? Are you willing to stand strong against the undermining effect of impatience on your long-term goals?

d) Use frugality.

In the early stages of your wealth creation, practice frugality. This doesn't mean being stingy or miserly, it means focusing on what you have and fully enjoying it. Then neediness will not drive you to impulsive spending. The modest lifestyle of frugality will enable you to control your spending in the early stages of wealth creation and so move you forward to the next stages.

e) Look for bargains.

To spend intelligently, decide to look for bargains, look for ways to save, learn how to use coupons to reduce expenses. If that seems below you dignity, then the issue of snobbery. That attitude will undermine your success. Refuse to let snobbery dig a grave of debt for you. Refuse to be seduced by promises of "Low Payments." Pay off all credit cards, refuse to live "on credit."

f) Stop all impulsive spending.

Impulsive spending is the destructive power that starts the downward spiral of debt creation. Refuse to impulsively and unthinkingly spend. It dis-empowers your financial strength. If you have to, get rid of your credit cards and don't carry much cash with you, nor your checkbooks. In other words, make it more difficult to quickly and easily pay for things. In this way you give yourself a chance to more fully consider your purchases instead of buying on impulse.

g) Distinguish between good and bad debt.
The basic principle is that the more people you are indebted to and that you have to pay, the poorer you are. That's how the debt game works. Kiyosaki recommends an entirely new principle about debt. He says that when you take on debt and risk, you should be paid for it. And how do you do that? Investing in a house as a rental property would be one way to do that. You provide the housing that someone else pays for and in the process, they pay the mortgage. So what is good debt versus bad debt? With good debt, you are enriched, your overall value is enhanced. "Bad" debt is what deletes all your resources.

5) Become a serious saver.
Your ability to create wealth has much less to do with how much you make (your income), than with *how much you save.* Salary, in fact, is actually one of the poorest indicators of financial success. Don't be seduced by salary. The question is how much do you save? How much can you save? Start with 10% of each paycheck and learn how to save, to build up capital.

An absolutely shocking statistic from the research of Machtig and Behrends (1997) is that there are as many CEOs living paycheck to paycheck as there are secretaries (p. 35). This highlights that the key is not the amount of your salary as much as it is how much are you saving. If your expenses are at the level of your income, you may have the look of wealth. It will not, however, be the reality. You may very well be only a paycheck or two away from having to move or declare bankruptcy. Clements (1989):

> "All the planning in the world isn't worth squat if you don't save. You won't have anything if you don't save. Refuse all of your excuses. The grim reality is, many folks never become serious savers. They squander money and time on purchases they don't even remember." (p. 17)

How to save?
1) Track your expenses.
To be able to spend less than you make, you have to know how much you spend and on what. A great many people amble

through life with absolutely no idea where the money goes, and never think of tracking their spending habits for a few months to see how they spend. Yet you can't control what you don't know or monitor. *Do you have your spending under your control?* If not, then make that your first priority.

Until you control your spending, you will probably fall victim to thinking that you need to get more and more. Track every dollar you spend to discover your patterns of consuming and waste. Do you have a budget? When will you develop your budget?

"Most people who build wealth in America are hard working, thrifty, and not at all glamorous. Wealth is rarely gained through the lottery, with a home run, or in quiz show fashion. But these are the rare jackpots that the press sensationalizes. Many Americans, especially those in the under accumulator of wealth category, don't know how to deal with increases in their realized income. They spend them! Their need for immediate gratification is great." (Stanley and Danko, p. 29)

2) Budget to save.

Begin by tracking everything you spend to discover your spending habits so that you can take control of them. Most people find this an incredible eye-opener. Save at least 10% of your pre-tax income. Use this to reduce your debt or to build up a capital fund.

3) Pay yourself first.

If creating wealth is a matter of how much you save and invest, not how much you earn, you will increase your financial wealth. Few do this. Few exercise the discipline to do it. Pay yourself first: write a check to your own "Investment Plan."

4) Only let assets buy luxuries.

While in the early stages, don't use your income to buy extras and luxuries, only the passive income of your assets.

5) Create a rainy day fund for liquid funds.

This will give you a sense of security and peace of mind. You can always find an excuse for not starting your Savings/ Investment program. Just do it. Do it systematically: regularly on the first of every month. Aim to create a fund that's equal in size to three months of pre-tax income; later you can increase that to the size of six months of pre-tax income.

6) Appreciate the power of accumulated interest.
Then there is the power of accumulated interest. Do you know about the value and importance of accumulated interest? $1 a day saved will grow to over $215,000 over 43 years at 10% interest which then provides $1400 a month income at retirement. $5 moves that up to more than $1,000,000.

*7) Learn how to **have** without **owning**.*
Do you know that you can *have* something—lots of things without needing to *own* them? It took me awhile to really get this one, but once I did, it has saved me lots and lots of money. The first time I really felt it was one day when I went to the public library while I was researching wealth creation. I found the desk that I always used, put my things there, and then went to the shelves to get some books. The shelves were full of books on the subject and suddenly it dawned on me:

> "All of these books are mine. *Mine!* I can come to my library and read my books anytime I want! And I don't even have to spend time working to maintain the books, the shelves, the building."

Later when I went for a run on the Colorado River Trail, I did so with new eyes, as I looked at the river, the trail, the woods, and the miles and miles of beautiful nature. "My running trail!" I was *having* without *owning*.

6) Learn how to increase your income.
There are many ways to increase your income. Use the following to begin stimulating your thinking about this. Access a state of playful creativity for brainstorming ideas.
    1) Write on a piece of paper ten of your favorite activities.
    2) Pick the top three of these that you would like to be paid for.
    3) Make a list of ten ways to provide some service or to create some product from what you love to do.
Are you willing to do what it takes to make money from the things you love to do? Then have some additional ways to discover and develop that:
    1) Find a way to give it away for awhile. Volunteer your services

to get experience.
2) Do it as a hobby.
3) Turn it into a side business out of your home.

Discover how to increase your income as an employee.
1) *Develop an engaged frame of mind.*
Assume for the next week that you own the business, that it is yours. Now walk around considering all the things you would do to improve things. How could I make it better, more efficient?

> **The Multiple Sources of Income Principle**
> Wealth is created through establishing a source of income from which to save and build to capital and from which to expand into multiple sources of income.

2) *Communicate your helpfulness.* Let the person or persons you report to know that you are on their side. Offer your ideas to your boss, supervisor, or manager and do so in the attitude that you are there to make them look good. As you do this, don't impose. Don't be a know-it-all, just offer it as a possible idea and give it away to them. If your attitude is one of truly caring and wanting to be helpful and you persist, it will eventually be recognized.

3) *Ask permission to do whatever needs to be done.* Take on smaller tasks. Develop the spirit of "going a second mile" above and beyond what you're paid for. Of course, this will require that you release all anger, bitterness, and resentment. It will require that you offer the very best attitude and spirit in your work. Do that for one month and see the difference it makes.

4) *Use an efficiency perspective.* Spend one week looking at things from the perspective of efficiency: How could I make things more efficient? Start with your own tasks. Learn how to do quality control for getting more and better results from your work.

5) *Develop a reputation for being a hard worker.* When you are at work, give yourself to actually working all the time you are there. Come in and give 10 extra minutes. Develop an identity as someone who others can depend on for getting things done and who does things effectively.

Discover ways to increase your income when you are self-employed.
1) Appreciate self-employment.

> One big danger for self-employed people is to feel small and inadequate and to feel limited by lack of capital, resources, people, etc. Yet these thoughts and feelings will only undermine your effectiveness. So chase away and refuse such negative attitudes. Write down at least ten values and blessings for being self-employed.

2) Take ownership of your business.

> Suppose you were to take complete ownership of your business, what would that mean for you and what would it lead you to do? What difference would it make if you dubbed yourself as the Owner?

3) Search for your value-add secret.

> Do you currently have a frame of mind that searches for how to add value to your customers? What do you need to change or shift so that value-adding becomes your dominant frame of mind? What value can you add to your customers? And what other value? How many values can you add?

The Frugality Principle:
Wealth is created in the early stages by using the delight of frugality. Wealth itself is the experience of

4) Learn to sell yourself and your ideas more effectively.

> Are you willing to learn how to increase your skills at selling yourself and your ideas?

Joyful Frugality as a Key to Getting Started

The first chapter in *The Millionaire Next Door* is entitled: *"Frugal, Frugal, Frugal."* Why? What does that mean? How could it be that important?

"Frugal" from the Latin root (*frug;* virtue; *frux;* fruit or value, and *frui;* to enjoy or have the use of). *Frugality is enjoying the virtue of getting good value* for every minute of your life energy and from everything you have the use of.

To explain frugality, Dominguez puts it in terms of your use and enjoyment of your possessions:

> "If you have ten dresses but still feel you have nothing to wear, you are probably a spendthrift. But if you have ten dresses and have enjoyed wearing all of them for years, you are frugal. Waste lies not in the number of possessions, but in the failure to enjoy them."

> "To be frugal means to have *a high joy-to-stuff ratio*. If you get one unit of joy for each material possession, that's frugal. But if you need ten possessions to even begin registering on the joy meter, you're missing the point of being alive. The Spanish word, *approvechar*, means to use something wisely—be it old zippers from worn-out clothing, or a sunny day at the beach. It's getting full value from life, enjoying all the good that each moment, and each thing has to offer. It's a succulent world, full of sunlight and flavor." (p. 167)

High joy-to-stuff-ratio! Full value ... enjoying all the good ... these are the words that describe frugality. Is that surprising? It is for many. In this, frugality not only enables you to get started, eliminate debt, and begin to build capital by saving, frugality also builds your financial intelligence. Frugality, as both an attitude and a set of actions, can enable you to align all aspects of your financial life with your values. To explain how frugality does that Dominguez writes:

> **The Financial Intelligence Principle:** *Wealth is created by developing financial intelligence.*
>
> That's because "A fool and his money is soon parted."

> "Financial independence is anything that frees you from a *dependence* on money to handle your life."

How to be Frugal
1) Decide to use frugality as a wealth creation strategy.
> Stanley and Danko discovered in their 1996 research seven common denominators among those who successfully build wealth. They said that the first is that the highly successful "live well below their means, they live with frugality."
>> "Being frugal is the cornerstone of wealth-building. ... We have to resist being seduced by a high-consumption lifestyle" (p. 23)
>
> This explains why the researchers said that the three words that profile the affluent are "frugal, frugal, frugal." (p. 28). Refuse to be seduced by things and consumption.

2) Accept restraint in spending.

"Whatever your income, always live below your means." (p. 161).

"To be frugal is to practice moderation, restraint, prudence, thrift, and financial equilibrium, but it certainly isn't being miserly or stingy. The rich get richer by acting poorer. The poor get poorer by acting richer." (Machig & Behrend)

3) Think in terms of resources.

Webster defines frugal as "characterized by or reflecting economy in the expenditure of resources." Frugality enables you to economize, to make good use of your resources and to not needlessly waste such. And not surprisingly, Stanley and Danko found that—

"... millionaires are frugal when frugality translates into real increases in the economic productivity of a household."

> **The Capitalizing Principle:**
> Wealth is created by saving and investing. It's not how much you earn that counts as much as how much you save. To build wealth you have to save money so that you can create and then invest Capital. Wealth is created by consistent saving.

4) Buy Quality.

The self-made millionaires are frugal about time expenditures, they distinguish between "first-cost" and life-cycle-cost. *They think in life-cycle distinctions.* So if you are buying cheap, you're probably not being frugal. Being frugal does not mean being cheap or miserly, it is *getting high value* for money and *enjoying it fully.* Stanley (2000) wrote:

"Most millionaires look to the future. They are very likely to compute the lifetime costs and benefits of various activities that have some potential in saving money. This type of behavior is a high correlation for accumulating wealth, and it's just one such element in the millionaires' overall frugal game plan." (p. 278)

5) Exercise the self-discipline to check numbers.

Donald Trump once cashed a check for 50 cents. It happened when *Spy* magazine ran an article, "Who is the Cheapest Millionaire." They sent out checks for 50 cents to see who would cash them. Trump did. His response?

> "They may call it cheap; I call it watching the bottom line. Every dollar counts in business, and for that matter, every dime. Penny-pinching? You bet, I'm all for it. I always try to read my bills to make sure I'm not being over-charged." (p. 59). "My parents hammered frugality into me at an early age, and it's the most important money-management skill a person can use. Call it penny-pinching if you want to; I call it financial smarts." (p. 61)

Figure 6:4

Liabilities	Assets
Intangible things:	
Internal: Stresses that drain, deplete	**Internal:** States that enrich
Tangible things:	

So, watch the bottom line. Do your books. Create and follow your budget to get your finances in order.

6) Distinguish Actual Assets and Liabilities
Frugality is also developed as you learn how to truly distinguish your assets from your liabilities. In handling your money, it's important to be able to distinguish assets and liabilities. An true "investment" is something that increases in value over time. If your investment loses value, it's not really an investment. It is a liability. The key is to remember that merely calling a purchase an "investment" doesn't make it so. When you buy things that cost to maintain and that decrease in value, you have *a liability* on your hands—and typically this means your

cars, boats, toys, computers, etc. Everything you buy that costs more than it produces increases your "cost of living." Yes, it may be necessary for your work— a car to drive to work, a computer to use, etc., yet these are still costs, not investments. It is a decreasing-in-value tool, not an increasing-in-value investment.

Examine what it costs you to maintain something in terms of the additional expenses, the responsibilities you accept, the mental-emotional involvement that are your true values, assets, and investments? Mind your true business by first distinguishing your *profession* and your *true investments.* What is your business? What are you doing that's creating assets? And to make maximum use of your assets, invest in things which go up in value. Kiyosaki asks rhetorically, "Is a banker's business banking?" And, of course, the answer is, "No. It's not unless he owns the bank."

My Personal Story
When I found myself back to zero in 1988, I knew that I was starting over again in terms of building financial stability. At the time the only wealth creation step that I had developed was the skill of saving. And I was a serious saver. And that's what had allowed me to buy my first house. Then in 1988 at 38 years of age and with all of the equity I had built up gone, I used frugality in a much more focused way to support my dream of financial stability.

While savings and capital did not allow the purchase of the second house, my growing understanding of wealth and how it is created did. I didn't know much, but I knew the difference between throwing money away in rent and investing it in my own real estate. So that's how I got started.

My next big decision was about self-investment. I knew that I needed more marketable skills— skills that would enable me to truly add value to others and solve problems. And having come across NLP in 1986 and having spent 1987 reading everything that was printed on NLP, I had begun to integrate NLP into my work. And doing so made me aware that this was the first self-investment that I would do.

As I then realized that if I was to be serious about it, I needed to invest in my training. That's what I did. The first training cost $3,000 at that time. And at that time it was 24 days long, and that meant closing my psychotherapy practice for nearly a month, and traveling more than a thousand miles west to San Diego. That's what I did. So the cost was more at $5,000, and while that would have been an acceptable debt because it would enable me to increase in my value to others, I decided to pay for it as I went. So I took my time, learning and practicing the models and saving up money for the next level.

One thing I enjoyed was learning, and that I learn best by writing, by making notes. It was that skill that I used when I took my original NLP notes. And from that came my first NLP book. How you ask? Discovering the value of NLP, when I took the master practitioner course, I brought my lap-top and a printer with me. Each day I took 4 to 5 pages of notes and each evening I printed them off so that I could review them. Pm day four, several participants noticed that I had notes on the training and asked about them, "Where did you get those notes?" I wrote them. The next question was always the same, "Can I get a copy of them?"

And yes, they could. By day ten, there were 40 pages, so I asked for some money to make copies of the notes, enough to pay for the paper and the printing. Later Richard Bandler heard about my notes and sent word through Beverly, the manager of NLP Products and Promotions that he wanted to talk to me. Several people warned me that I was in trouble now! But that wasn't my attitude. When I went to the penthouse to see Richard, it turned out that he also liked them. So much so, in fact, that he invited me to return to Trainers Training the following year to write the notes for that training as well.

Fast forward several years, and having cleaned up the notes, added details to them, I sent them off to *Crown House Publications* only to get a call directly from Dr. Martin Roberts, the publisher. He wanted to print the notes as a book, which he did. Today that book is *The Spirit of NLP* (1996). And, guess what? It still brings in revenue.[1]

Your Adventure in Creating Wealth
As your Wealth Coach let me whisper a secret in your ear—for most people *getting started* is the hardest step of all. It's the inertia thing. It is much easier to keep moving once you are moving. The hardest part is pushing yourself to get going in the first place. Is that true for you? The danger at this point is asking yourself the "why" question: "Why am I this way?" If that is your temptation to any extent, *Do not do that!*

Avoid that at all costs! It will only send you into psycho-archeology and imprison you in a pit of self-pity and victimhood.

The truth is —it doesn't matter why you have not started or why you are that way, or why you find it hard to start. *Just start!* Just do it. Forget all of the mental philosophizing about inertia. That only feeds inertia.

The question to ask yourself is *the resource question:*
> What do you need in order to get started? What do you need to do, think, or feel? What would get you going even if there's some negative emotions?

Given that I've offered you many practical steps in this chapter for beginning, what will be your first step? Take a few minutes to go back through the pages of this chapter and choose what would make the most transformative difference for you.
- Where would you like to devote your time this week in getting started?
- Do you need to adjust your thinking, believing, and attitude?
- Do you need to work out your budget?
- Do you need to access a more effective work state?

Now make a list of things under the following categories:
- What self-investment do you need to make?
- Where and in what way can frugality assist you in your wealth creation plan?
- Make a list of your assets and liabilities. Revisit it every day for a week until you have it fully filled out.

End of Chapter Notes:
1. *The Spirit of NLP* (1996) published by Crown House Publications, see www.crownhouse.co.uk.

Chapter 7

HOW DO *I* CREATE WEALTH?

The Engine of Wealth Creation

"We are born to grow rich through the use of our faculties."
Ralph Waldo Emerson

"No man is free who is not a master of himself."
Epictetus

In principle, you now know *how* to create wealth, do you not? And how do you or anyone else create wealth?
You use your skills and expertise to create valuable products and services that add value to people.

Do that and people will pay for what you can do for them. It's as simple as that. That's how you do it in principle. *Yet how do you specifically do it?* What skills do you have for creating wealth? What expertise? What specific products and services will you create and what specific problems will you solve? It's now time to get down to specifics—which is the focus and purpose of this chapter.

It's About the Right Job
Are you in the perfect job for you for creating wealth? Are you in the most perfect job that ideally fits your talents, skills, interests, and passions? Do you totally and absolutely care about what you do? How passionate are you about it? Are you willing to become passionate about

it? Are you willing to find a job you are fit to do, give yourself to it, learn to love it, and honor the actions that make it enriching?

This was another of the surprising discoveries of the wealth researchers. They discovered that those who got rich and who created the most wealth were *those who found jobs that they loved.* And they said that their jobs felt more like "a calling" to them than a job. It was their love and passion. Their job served as their economic engine—the mechanism that generated their money.

Stanley and Danko (1996) discovered that the self-made millionaires somehow "chose the right occupation." And for that reason 86% of self-made millionaires said that they actually *love* their work (p. 62).
> "If you want to be successful, select a vocation you love. It's amazing how well people do in life when their vocation is one that stimulates dedication and positive emotions." (p. 65)

And in his second book, Stanley (2000) concluded that you need to find a business you can love—a career that allows you to make full use of your abilities and aptitudes. If you select the wrong vocation, you are more likely to grow to dislike it which is a big mistake. And so in a chapter with the title, *Vocation, Vocation, Vocation,* he writes that "If you are creative enough to select the ideal vocation, you can win, win big-time." This means that the bedrock of the ideal vocation is—
> "You love the products you produce. You have affection for your customers and suppliers." (pp. 19, 21)
>
> "The key is to find the job that's well suited to your talents, and then it's easier to fall in love with it. But you should also find one that has the potential to make you rich. If you account for these factors, you'll be amazed at how well disciplined you become. Time and work hours pass quickly when you're having fun." (p. 213)
>
> "As most millionaires report, stress is a direct result of devoting a lot of effort to a task that's not in line with one's abilities. It's more difficult, more demanding mentally and physically, to work in a vocation that's unsuitable to your aptitude." (p. 220)
>
> "Some of the activities your work now forces you to overlook may be the very ones you'd find most absorbing. And inasmuch as no one else is paying you to do them, you will have to pay yourself for doing them." (p. 93)

Similarly, Martha Sinetar concludes that it is *goodness of fit* between your skills, interests, passions, your daily tasks, and your means of livelihood that is the secret of wealth creation. Sinetar speaks about this as "the beauty of right livelihood."

> "As people honor the actions they value most—by *doing* them they become more authentic, more reliable, more self-disciplined. They grow to trust themselves more; they learn to listen to their own inner voice as a steady, truthful and strengthening guide for what to do next and even how to do it." (p. 5)

Choosing a Job You Can Love

If a key ingredient of wealth creation is selecting the right task, vocation, or job, then how do you do that? How can you find it sooner rather than later? What processes can enable you to discover a value that you could create that could become your economic engine for wealth? There are several questions you can ask to begin to discover what's best for you.[1]

First, explore your basic attitude.
How much do you like your present job? Do you love it? Do you enjoying doing what it is that you do? Could you? The more you love and enjoy your work, the more you will lose track of time and the more you become absorbed in the value-creating activity itself.

The evidence points overwhelmingly that *work you enjoy is far more likely to make you rich than any investment*. Actually, this gives you two forms of wealth: first the enjoyment of work and second, financial success from the work. After all, only by being quietly captivated will make you persist through any and every obstacle. And if you don't love it, could you? Do you need to change your attitude? Do you need to learn the skill of giving yourself to something so that you learn to love it?

Second, explore your basic talents, gifts, and dispositions.
Are you a natural fit for the job that you want? Who is? What are the inescapable requirements for that job? When you test yourself using the Multiple Intelligence (MI) questions and distinctions, what shows up as your natural strengths and dispositions? (See a list of MI questions in the box at the end of this chapter.)

Inside-out wealth begins from the "wealth" you develop within yourself —within your mind-body-emotion system. It comes from your powers, that is, from your "ability to act effectively and efficiently" (which is what "power" refers to). So, what can you do now that creates value?

What can you learn to do that will create value for others? The richer your ability or power to act, the richer your choices and ability to create wealth for which you will then be rewarded. And this again explains why you first have to develop your inner powers and personal subjective sense of wealth. Your inner resourcefulness enables your creativity and therefore your ability to use your potentials to create value.

The Art of Passion Finding

There are two ways to identify a passion that you can then use for your wealth creation engine. You can either find it or create it.

1) *Finding your passion.*
Find your passion inside of your dreams, talents, hopes, dispositions, skills, etc. Take any one of these words and use it to discover the passions you have within. Then as you find your talents, transform them into passions by patiently and mindfully developing them. After all, even talents have to be developed and connected to a trade by which you can create values for others in the marketplace.

2) *Creating your passion.*
Create your passion from you abilities, interests, and opportunities. What activities could you fall in love with or become absorbed in? What happens if you think about your work as "an expression of your love?" While it is true, as Sinetar says, that if you do what you love "the money will follow," by itself that statement is incomplete and can be misleading. We can easily adjust this statement to make it more accurate by saying:
> Do what you love which is market-able and adds value to others (a value that others want or need and will pay for), and the money will follow.

Talent Search

If each of us can create wealth by playing to the strength of our talents, how are you doing with this? Have you discovered your core strengths and talents? Do you know them? Have you discovered how to use your talents to create financial wealth? If not, then is it time to go on a talent search—to discover what talents to develop, what knowledge to learn, what skills to master, and what market to apply them to?

Begin by using the SWOT analysis questions to explore yourself and your life situation. Use the questions in the box on the next page. As you go through the questions, use them to explore your talents. And as you find them, make a list of your talents and strengths. Next, begin to separate out a *passionate talent* along with your core and supportive skills. What are you passionate about? What makes you feel more fully alive?

Of course, finding a passionate talent isn't enough. Next brainstorm a dozen ways to make money from the talent.

> How could you make money from this talent? Who would pay you for applying and using this talent? What value would they receive from the application of your talent? What benefits would accrue to them? Does it suit your aptitudes? Does your attitude support it?

As you identify your strengths and weaknesses, meta-question each one in order to find your singularity. That is, meta-question your beliefs, understandings, decisions, meanings, identities, etc. about what you discover. This will reveal your higher frames that embed these strengths and weaknesses. What interaction have you found between your potentials and your passions? How can you combine your passion with an economic engine that will create profit?

The Irritation Index
Do you still not know your passion? Then let's use your irritation as a feeling for finding your way forward. And why would you do that? How does that help? Do this because when you go to work, you are paid to *not* be doing some things so that you can do what the job requires. Now, do you find that irritating? How much does that irritate you? You are irritated because you would rather be doing what? Where would you rather be and rather be doing?

This gives you something else to explore. If searching for the bright side of your passions don't produce the results you want, explore the dark side of your irritations. So go to work for the next month, and during your breaks and lunch hour, entertain this sentence and complete it with as many sentence completions as possible: *"What I'd rather be doing is..."* When you complete two dozen sentence completions, then work on this one: *"If I had all the money I wanted, what I would be doing to fulfill my potential skills is..."*

As you let your mind go to these places, massage it in your mind. What would be a "good job" for you? What would be a great job? What would you be doing? With whom? What would be your objective?

The Art of Passion Creation

If you don't know and don't seem to be able to find your passion, then another option is to *create* it. What would you *like* to become passionate about? What talents, skills, interests, likes, etc. would you like to develop a passion for?

First, begin by identifying an area that has possibility for good financial rewards. What skills would you have to develop? Make a list. What knowledge base would you have to learn? Make a list. Who do you know that is successful in this area? Identify some skillful people in this area to interview.

Next, create a plan for moving forward. How much time are you willing to devote to this area for learning and skill development? Create a plan to fit that time-frame.

> *"Interest" is interesting.*
> The word literally refers to existing (*est*) within (*inter*) something. You take interest in something when you put yourself into it.

When you have your plan in place, now enter into the Matrix of that passion.[2] What beliefs, understandings, meanings, decisions, etc. would create more interest and passion in this area? What else? How can you more fully *enter into* (inter-est) this subject or area? Are you fully willing to interest yourself in this? What intention would support this? What higher intention? What would be the highest intention?

As you now step back from this possibility, are you willing to persist in this? Are you willing to invest more time and effort into this? How much? What beliefs would support your persistence? What else?

If so, then set a commitment for developing and creating a passion. What level of commitment are you willing to invest? What beliefs would support your commitment? What decision would support it? Anchor and future pace your passion creation.
What would be a good anchor for this state? How aligned are you with this at this point in time?

SWOT Analysis

Strengths: *Advantages*
    What are your talents and natural dispositions?
    What are your core competencies and proven skills?
    What can you or do you uniquely offer?
    What expertise have you developed over the years?
    What are your passions and interests?
    What do you love doing?
    What supporting skills will you need?

Weaknesses: *Dis-advantages*
    What are your weaknesses?
    Where are you deficit of critical talents or skills?
    What do you need to do to manage these weaknesses?
    How can you and will you handle them so they do not undermine your strengths?
    What hurts, pains, humiliations, and even traumas have you experienced and found a solution, to or could find a solution?
    What hurt in life has put a searching question in you?
    What hurt have you been through that gives you special insights about that problem and its solution?

Opportunities:
    What opportunities do you see before you?
    What circumstances could you use as an opportunity?
    What problems or needs do you have a passion to address?
    What do you really care about — passionately?
    What do you love doing?

Threats:
    What factors might impact negatively on you and your situation?
    What changes or stresses threaten or upset you?
    What threats could unleash potentials that are yet untapped within you?

Your Wealth Singularity

In his best selling book, *Good to Great,* Jim Collin describes a process for a company or business to identify what that organization can focus on in order to be the best in the world. He speaks of it as a singularity—a singularity that arises from the interface of three variables. Those three variables are potential, passion, and profit. At the point where the three come together— a firm can identify its best possibility for becoming a great company.

We can equally apply these three variables to ourselves. To find your singularity, find the interface of these same three variables:

Potential: What you are uniquely wired and predisposed to do, what fits your unique gifts and talents. This is the importance of your talent search for what you can become highly skilled in doing that could add value to others. If you didn't do the SWOT analysis, do that now as part of your talent search.

Passion: The meanings about an activity that make it valuable, significant, and inspirational. Your passion is a result of your thinking, understanding, interpretive style, and meaning-making ability. This is what you worked on as you sought to either find or create your passion.

Profit: Your vehicle for making money is the economic engine that fits the demands of your culture and what people will pay for. Next, develop a business plan that identifies the numbers that can make a business succeed.

Finding your singularity will be at the intersect point of your highest meanings (passion) and your best skills (performance). When these combine in the context of your work, vocation, career, and the current market, you have your singularity. If you then focus on it, become absorbed in it, and become utterly fascinated by it you will find the wealth creation fairly easy.

Identifying and Meta-Stating your Singularity

Do you know your singularity? Have you identified it yet? If so, what is your singularity? What opportunities do you see that you will be seizing?

Yet knowing your singularity is not enough, you have to act on it and that will require the strength of several key states and strategies. Among the most important are the following. As you read down

through this list, gauge how strong you are in these states from 0 to 10:
- ___ Courage to take action
- ___ Proactive
- ___ Persistence
- ___ Resilience
- ___ Efficiency
- ___ Fun/ playful as you work
- ___ Self-efficacy

Figure 7:1

THE SINGULARITY

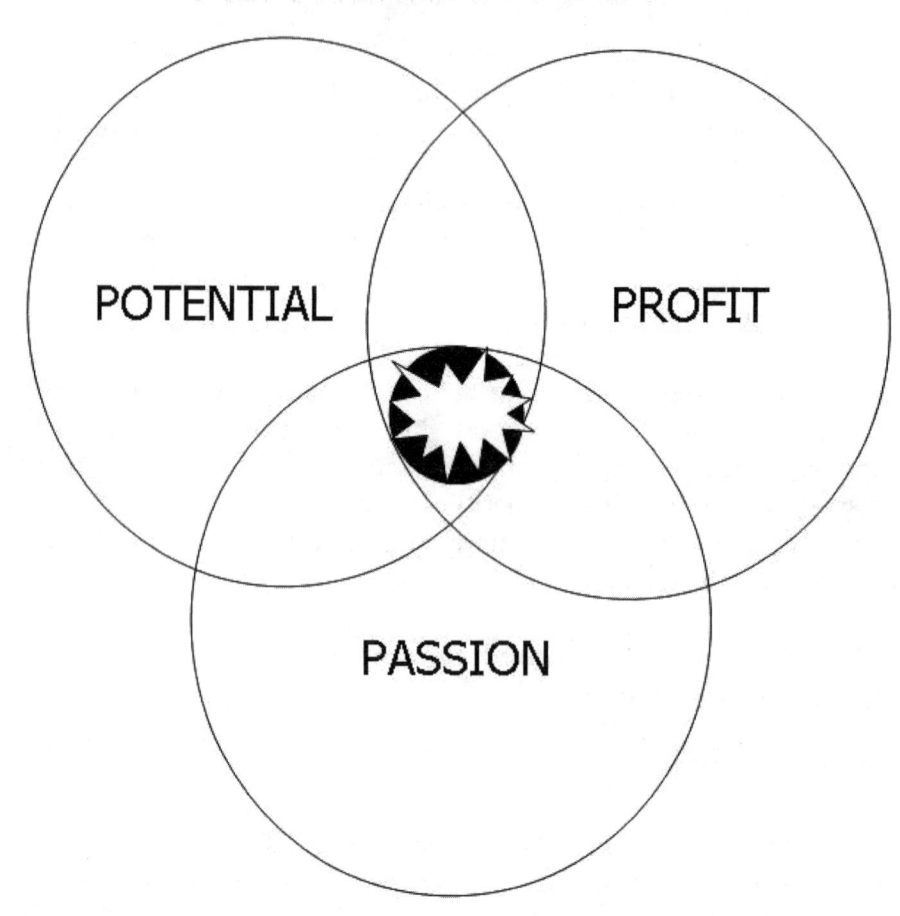

POTENTIAL   PROFIT

PASSION

Do you have the requisite states to tap into the potentials of your singularity? If you were to address one of them right now, which of these would create the most leverage for you? This will identify your key leverage point for empowerment.

Undermining the Synergy of Your Passion and Potential
If finding your wealth creation singularity begins here and if there are ways to find and/or develop a passion from your potential gifts and talents, then what could stop you? What could prevent you from effectively identifying your singularity?

The central thing that could sabotage your singularity is *losing interest.* Have you ever lost interest in something? Of course you have, we all have. So how did that happen? What contributes to this devastating experience of "losing interest?"

Typically it occurs through frustrations—things not working out, disappointment due to unrealistic expectations, having to deal with lots of trivial and petty details, disliking and spending a lot of energy complaining about all of the stupid things you have to put up with, snobbery that invites contempt of the small details or a job "beneath your dignity." What frustrates you? How much frustration-tolerance do you have?

Low frustration-tolerance is a factor that downgrades your "interest." If you give in to it, in the end you will lose interest in that possibility. Such low tolerance of frustration is typically tied to rigid ideas about the way things "should" be. So if you put "shoulds" on things—demand that things be a certain way, that you *should* get what you want when you want it, you thereby lower your tolerance level. You create *a demanding-ness* that will increase your state of discontent, dislike, contempt, annoyance, and irritation. And all of this will lower your ability to handle frustrations.

When you have all of this in place, it doesn't take much to lower your interest in something. The demanding-ness, the shoulds, and the rigid expectations will puncture your passion and interest causing you to "lose interest," your wealth creation potential will evaporate.

Becoming the CEO of Your Singularity
While the phrase "self-discipline" is typically a turn-off for most people,

the idea is not. Inside the word *self-discipline there* is a great idea. So what is the idea? Self-discipline means mastering yourself so that you can get yourself to actually *do* what you want to do. Isn't that an attractive, compelling, and desirable idea? With self-discipline you are in charge of you! With self-discipline you possess an internal compass, a control and navigational system that keeps you on track.

And what does it feel like to take control of your potential and passion and specific profit mechanism? What do we call that? We use such words as self-discipline, self-control, and self-mastery.

For the ability to create wealth and business success, Robert Allen emphasizes that "control is essential." Self-discipline and self-initiation enable you to get yourself to *do* what you know you want to and need to do. As a disciplined person you will then not be easily sidetracked from your vision and mission.

> "If you're willing to do only what's easy, life will be hard. But if you are willing to do what's hard, life will be easy."
> Harv Eker (2005, p. 169)

- How well do you discipline yourself to do the things that you need to do?
- How much self-initiation do you have?
- How well do you plan, budget, save, enrich your business knowledge?

Are you ready to take ownership of your financial destiny? Are you ready to refuse to blame or whine? Are you ready to fully acknowledge, "It's in my hands." This requires that you be proactive rather than reactive or defensive and refuse to be pushed around by problems or emotions.

> "If you can't master the power of self-discipline, it is best not to try to get rich."
> Kiyosaki (p. 164)

Discipline emerges when you learn how to take control of yourself —of your mind and your body.[3] You need discipline because even the very best financial plans will be totally ineffective *if you don't follow through.* It takes discipline to become affluent, it takes the discipline to budget, save, and control expenditures.

> "Most people *want* to be physically fit. And the majority know what is required to achieve this. Yet despite that knowledge, most people never become well conditioned physically. Why not? Because they don't

have the discipline to just do it. They don't budget their time to just do it. It is like becoming wealthy in America." (Blotnick, p. 40)

Will you take full responsibility for your money and for investing it wisely? This means keeping it under your scrutiny and control. This translates to taking a proactive stance and continually monitor your investments.

Contrast all of this to those who lack self-discipline. Stanley and Danko (1996) describe some parents of the self-made first-generation millionaires as providing "economic outpatient care." This means that they constantly bailed them out from the consequences of their behaviors and failed to coach them to learn independence, self-reliance, and financial intelligence. If they had coached them, then their adult children would have become economically self-sufficient.

Self-Discipline or Luck
Another disorientation from following your passion is the mythology of getting a lucky break, the "big break" that suddenly solves all of your financial problems, and puts you in the ideal job or investment. But waiting for that disorients you from what you need to be doing to create wealth. Instead, focus on developing your ability to proactively respond to the opportunities that correspond to your natural skills and expertise.

Speaking about discipline brings up another myth and delusion to give up, namely, *getting rich without effort*. Those who are consistent winners in the realm of creating wealth are not deceived about that. They are always preparing. They prepare so that they are ready when an opportunity arise. They also prepare to see opportunities in the everyday problems that challenge them.

> "Wealth, like happiness, is never attained when sought after directly. It always comes as a by-product of providing a useful service."
> Henry Ford

Then when an opportunity does arise, when your competence and understanding tells you that there's a chance for you that may lead to wealth, you will not delay or procrastinate. Clawson (1926) wrote:
> "Good luck waits to come to that man who accepts opportunity." (p. 50)
> "Risk is the price you pay for opportunity." (Robert Allen)

If you are unprepared, then you will never see or respond to what we call "good luck," or the opportune moment. Luck flees from those given to procrastination and fear. Give up needless delaying when you know that something is a good choice. Actually, you can increase your ability to attract good luck to yourself by preparing, learning your trade, and knowing your criteria for what fits for your values and situation. Then when opportunity arises, you'll be ready and able to take advantage of the opportunity.

Initiation — a Step of Discipline
Part of self-discipline is the ability to push yourself. Blotnick (1980) noted this in his research:
> "We often have to push ourselves a bit to get started before the enjoyment takes over and carries us the rest of the way. Both people who succeeded and those who failed often required an initial boost to get going. The two groups differed significantly in their *willingness to give themselves* that needed first push. (p. 101)

He noted that those who eventually became millionaires "displayed an ability to get themselves moving, in spite of an initial reluctance to do so." They accepted that there is usually a warming up phase in achieving anything. Blotnick described this as a "thought-and-image-gathering phase" and noted that they would use it to get themselves into doing whatever needed to be done.

Those who failed said things like, "If I don't feel like doing it, maybe I really don't want to." Taking counsel of their dis-comfort, they would then hold back. In doing so, they train themselves to *not* take effective action. This description identifies the strength of heart in people who are self-disciplined to do difficult things. Being response-able, they make "hard" decisions as they say *yes* to what they want and *no* to good choices. In this they can say a definite *yes* to the best choices.

To *not* do something that needs to be done because you don't feel like doing it is a recipe for failure. The problem here is the interpretation. To interpret that a feeling of reluctance means that you lack the interest, or that you shouldn't do it, or shouldn't force yourself to do it, that interpretation destroys your motivation. The problem is *the meaning* you give to a feeling. You then perform that meaning by avoiding the required activities. No wonder this is a recipe for failure.

My Personal Story

It actually took me a really, really long time before I discovered my singularity. In terms of potentials, I think it began when I took "typing" as a class in the ninth grade. I was a natural with the typing. When I completed the class, I was typing sixty-words a minute. Being highly kinesthetic I remember running the "typing" patterns with my fingers as I imagined typing all day long. Perhaps that's why I developed typing skills as quickly as I did.

Then there was the experience of learning by writing. For years I didn't even know it was happening. But in high school, and then in college, I "naturally" found myself writing in order to understand. Friends and others often told me that I was wasting time and effort, "Just read it aloud!" they would say. Or they would say, "Write an outline." But what came more naturally, and what drove the learnings home for me, was writing about whatever I was studying.

My first career was in ministry and I had a mentor even before going to college. I grew up in a conservative Protestant church and a local minister had initiated a training program for promising young men. He helped me with public speaking and memorizing texts and so off I went to "save the world, one soul at a time." The experience seemed to fit and called forth a natural passion to help people. Why? I think because of the "problem" that I experienced when I was a young teenager with my mother when she was taken from the family and committed to a mental hospital. I didn't understand that; and no one explained it to me. So it left a not-knowing-what-was-going-on gap in me which generated an intense curiosity about people. "Why do such things happen to people and what can help them?" So while still teenager, I connected helping with the ministry. And also being rash, impulsive, and impatient off I took! [You can find the full story in *Unleashed,* 2007.]

All seemed to be going pretty good while I was in school, but as soon as I graduated and took a church as a young minister, problems began. During the first five years I got fired every twelve-months—year after year until I finally "got it." I was too radical—I was asking too many questions. I upset too many people. I push too hard and I had too much of a disturbing style. My interest was actually in helping people cope with life, not defend an intellectual creed

The last firing put me back to zero in terms of career and it didn't take long to discover that a Master's Degree in Biblical Language and Literature with a focus on ancient Greek and Hebrew on my resume didn't make any points or impress anyone! Oops. And with the firings, loss of income, alienation of friends, *I* needed therapy! And that began an intensive study of psychology— Freud, Jung, Adler, T.A., Ellis' Rational-Emotive, etc. And that led to getting certificates in various forms of psychotherapy and eventually to opening my own Counseling Practice.

My passion was now in full blossom—still trying to understand people—myself first, and then others. And as I did, I was reading and writing, and so using literature was a natural way I sought to help others. Eventually it sent me back to school. I first wanted a business degree because I had learned that lesson, so I got a Bachelor of Science in Human Resources; then as I saved money and returned to school, a Master's in Clinical Psychology, and finally a Ph.D. in Cognitive-Behavioral Psychology.

While caught up in those studies and having begun conducing Communication Trainings, I happened upon the field of NLP. That led me to begin reading Bateson, Korzybski, and many other seminal thinkers. Fast forward a few years later, and I stumbled onto the idea of meta-states which, in turn, lead me to developing the Meta-States Model.

So what was my passion?
> Helping people, making a difference, enabling and empowering people to cope well, to master life's challenges, and to find the meaning of things. And to do all of that, reading and writing to find the most powerful tools for that kind of empowerment.

And my potentials?
> Reading, writing to learn, curiously searching and questioning, testing things pragmatically to identify what actually works and what doesn't.

What was the "profit" part of my singularity? What was the economic engine I used to create wealth?
> Research leading to practical literature, books, training manuals within the self-development, self-actualization fields of cognitive-behavioral psychology and NLP and eventually developing

Neuro-Semantics for launching a new human potential movement.

Your Adventure in Creating Wealth
Coaching time again. Now you know that one of the key secrets is "vocation, vocation, vocation." Now you know that wealth is created by finding the right job, and finding a fit between your talents and passions. So where are you in terms of finding your perfect job? What gifts clamor within you for expression? Where do you naturally feel more alive and fascinated?

Take time this week to work through the SWOT questions and then the meta-SWOT questions to begin to identify your strengths.

After you do that, ask five people who know you very well what they consider your strengths and gifts. If wealth creation arises from the value that you create for others by means of the gifts that you have, then begin to make a list of all the values and benefits that you can offer others.

If you didn't do the sentence stem exercise under the section on "the Irritation Index," be sure to go back to that now and complete that section.

End of Chapter Notes
1. Harvard psychologist Howard Gardner mapped out a new model of intelligence in his books, *Frames of Mind* (1983), *The Unschooled Mind* (1991), *Multiple Intelligences* (1993), *etc.* This initiated a new movement in education by expanding the old definitions of "intelligence." Gardner views the mind as modular —each intelligence comes from a distinct portion of the brain that operates somewhat independently of the others. We do not just have "one intelligence," we have *multiple* intelligences. "Intelligence" is not a single or general capacity. It is the ability to solve problems, create products and responses that are valued and useful in a given context. "Intelligence" relates in a relative way to various domains or contexts as problem solving skills.

2. Matrix questions are meta-questions as well. There are seven categories for these meta-questions: meaning and intention, an then self, capacities (power), relationships (others), time, and world (universes of meaning).

3. They For a whole book on how to get yourself to follow-through, execute what you know, and implement your highest plans, see *Achieving Peak Performance* (2009). That book is all about closing the knowing–dong gap.

The Multiple Intelligence Model

1) Linguistic Intelligence
   Used in reading a book, writing a paper, novel, or poem; and understanding spoken words.

2) Logical-Mathematical Intelligence
   Used in solving mathematical problems, balancing a checkbook, doing a mathematical proof, and in logical reasoning.

3) Spatial Intelligence
   Used in getting from one place to another, in reading a map, and in packing suitcases in the truck of a car.

4) Musical Intelligence
   Used in singing a song, composing a sonata, playing a trumpet, or even appreciating the structure of a piece of music.

5) Bodily Kinesthetic Intelligence
   Used in dancing, playing basketball, running a mile, or throwing a javelin.

6) Inter-personal Intelligence
   Used in relating to other people, such as when we try to understand another person's behavior, motives, or emotions.

7) Intra-personal Intelligence
   Used in understanding ourselves— the basis for understanding who we are, what makes us tick, and how we can change ourselves, given the existing constrains on our abilities and interests.

Chapter 8

AM *I* A WEALTH CREATOR?

Wealth is ... "the ability to think well of ourselves and our abilities even without money."
                                    Martha Sinetar

During the past six or seven years I have received dozens of emails from people congratulating me on my work or asking me how it feels to know that I have created jobs for hundreds of people. The first time I received one of those questions, I immediately dismissed it. "Me? I didn't create any jobs." Eventually, however, I slowly came to realize that the models, patterns, and structures set up through the International Society of Neuro-Semantics has indeed provided jobs and income and wealth for many people. And that began to change my identity, "Hey I have created wealth for others! That means I'm a *Wealth Creator*."

I still remember when I first tried on that identity, "I'm a creator of wealth for myself and others." It felt strange, heady, and yet exciting. I liked it! I want to be a wealth creator. I want to make that kind of difference for others, to help many people find and release their wealth creation powers. How about you? Would you like to put *Wealth Creator* on your business card? Would you like to know yourself as someone who creates wealth for yourself and others?

Because *inside-out wealth* focuses first *within* and then *without* as you build rich and abundant states of mind-emotion, you don't need money to become rich or to become a "somebody." You create wealth more simply —as an expression of the value you create. How do you do this?

> **The Inside-Out Principle:**
> *Wealth is created from the inside out. You experience it first as an inward value that moves you to experience a rich state of mind-and-heart that enables you to make it real in the outside world as you create value for others.*

To do this requires several things. It requires that you do or create the following:

1) *Self-Esteem.* Esteem your self as unconditionally valuable to establish your inner wealth as a person.

2) *Self-Acceptance.* Accept your self in terms of what you have, what you do not have, your gifts, the gifts that you do not have, the life conditions that you find yourself in whether you like them or not.

3) *Self-Confidence.* Develop competencies from the gifts you do have in order to feel confident about what you can do and contribute, the difference you can make.

4) *Self-Efficacy.* Trust yourself for the competencies you will develop in the future, trust your ability to learn and develop the required skills.

5) *Self-Capitalization.* Capitalize on your best talents and highest visions to unleash your highest potentials.

6) *Self-Optimism.* Set boundaries on yourself with regard to creating "hurt" and/or "evil" from events so you operate from a core of optimism within.

7) *Self-Investment.* Invest in your ongoing development of mind, body, and emotions and embrace ambiguity to unleash your innate creativity.

8) *Self-Integrity.* Ground yourself in a self-integrity of living up to your highest values and visions, being a person of your word and trustworthy.

1) Self-Esteem[1]

All the money in the world will not make you worth more than you are right now. It will not make you more of a person, more of "a somebody," more important. It will not add to your value or self-esteem one bit. Do you know that? How firmly do you know that? If you don't solidly know that, you are in danger of mis-using money, in danger of trying to use money to bolster your self-esteem. And, because that is something money cannot do, it is unsane.

You are truly wealthy when you are not *dependent* on money for feeling good about yourself, for feeling important, significant, valuable, or rich. How well can you maintain these critical states without needing to "have" money? To that extent you are already "rich." Are you rich in all of your many facets of self?

The truth is that money does not, and cannot, increase your value as a person. It does not make you more important or a somebody. If you want money for these reasons, money will become a pathology—a neurotic need that will undermine your effectiveness.

Self-esteem is exactly that— *self*-esteem. *You* have to do it. You have to appraise or esteem yourself as a human being, as a person, as having innate and unconditional value. It means applying value and dignity to yourself as an unconditionally valuable human being with no need to prove yourself or do anything to become "a someone." You were born a somebody, were you not? Yes. And so is everybody else! Self-esteem is the ability to think well of yourself and your value or worth as a person and to do so apart from money and status symbols.

What does it take to *be* a wealth creator? What are the elements that come together making you a creator of wealth in all of its dimensions? *Being* wealth, which is the inside part of wealth creation, involves feeling yourself having worth and value. You don't have to *do* anything in order to *be* who and what you are— a human being. Worth as a person is given in the fact that you are a human being. Will you accept that that is enough to establish your worth and value?

2) Self-Acceptance

Once you esteem yourself with dignity and worth that is not conditioned on anything, then you can more easily move to self-acceptance. This means accepting and acknowledging yourself as you are. It means facing the facts of your existence, self, life, situation, gifts as what you have and have to deal with and to do so without falling apart. Martha Sinetar writes:
> "Until we accept ourselves, it is unlikely that our vocational uniqueness

will reveal itself through us, since vocation is nothing more than a way to live productively and uniquely." (p. 35)

Accepting self means accepting your strengths and your weaknesses, your potentials and the potentials that you do *not* have. It doesn't mean resigning or condoning your situation. It simply means acknowledging the cards that life has dealt you. The magic of acceptance is that it allows you to stop the fight. Acceptance ends the war. And when you do that, you will release lots of energy for effective action and creativity.

The opposite is self-rejection and self-contempt which are states that will sabotage your highest and best. And why reject yourself? Why show contempt to yourself? *Judgment.* You are judging yourself, your situation, your looks, gifts, etc. You are not treating yourself in a kind and gentle way, but you are harshly and cruelly "rating" your humanity in a way so that you come up short.

3) Self-Confidence

Being wealth leads to *doing* wealth—the outside part of wealth creation. This entails a different meta-state—the state of *self-confidence.* This refers to believing and trusting (*fideo*) in what you can *do.* Self-confidence relates to you as a *human doing* whereas self-esteem relates to being *a human being.* How can you convince the best people to work for you if they see self-doubt in your eyes? How can you sell anything? If you believe you can succeed, the probabilities are greatly enhanced that you will reach and even exceed your goals. Are you confident to forthrightly assert your vision, opinion and values, to stand up for yourself, to stand apart, to courageously follow your passions?

Self-confidence relates to your core competencies—to your potentials and passion—and so to your singularity. Yet self-confidence, unlike self-esteem, is conditional. It is conditioned upon your actual skills—upon developing your talents so that you become competent in what you do. Then you can take pride in what you can actualize and contribute. A particular danger here is that you will go after *the feeling* of confidence and neglect *the conditions* for the feeling—the required competency. So forget about *feeling* self-confident and focus on developing the competencies. The self-confident feelings will follow.

4) Self-Efficacy

Developing self-efficacy takes self-confidence to the next level— to a whole new dimension of experience. It moves you from the past to the future. That's because self-confidence depends on the past—on what you have *already proved* that you can do. So you feel confident that you are able to perform a particular skill. You are competent and you know it.

By contrast, self-efficacy is about the future. It is a belief in your capacity to learn, figure things out, and solve new problems. It is the conviction that you *can* always do something about whatever happens. It is the attitude: "No matter what happens, I will figure out how to cope, I will figure out a solution."

Because I have learned how to drive on both sides of the road, the right side in the United States and the left side in Australia and other formerly British countries, I am *confident* in myself and my ability to be able to do that. And because I have never piloted a plane, I have no confidence about that, no self-confidence. Yet I have the self-efficacy that I could pilot a plane. I could go for that and add that to my new learnings if I so chose or if it became important for some reason. My efficacy is based on my past confidences about taking on a new skill and being able to learn it.

Self-efficacy involves a greater sense of yourself. You have a greater sense of your powers than of the problems that you face. Begin by thinking of a problem that you have, a problem to your wealth creation. How big of a problem is it from 0 to 10? How big is the problem in your representations? How big are you in proportion to the problem? Which is bigger? How big do you need to be to handle the problem?
    A Level 5 problem
    A Level 2 you – Big problem!
    A Level 8 you — No problem! It would not even register as a problem in your brain.

Now you are ready to make yourself bigger (in your mind) than the problem. So grow yourself to be twice as big as the problem. The problem is not the size of the problem, it is your size in relation to the problem. So as you think about the problem— notice your internal representations of yourself and the problem. Which is bigger? What resources will make you bigger? How are you playing small? How can you turn that around and play bigger in the game? When you feel you have a big problem, and you are playing small, you are discounting your powers and potentials. If that's what you're going to do, then go ahead and point to yourself and scream out: "Mini me! Mini me! Mini me!" (Harv Eker)

Do that in various tones of voices until you burst out in laughter—feeling ridiculous and are ready to stop. Then swell up to your higher self, take a deep breath, float up, and as you decide to be bigger than the problem, become much bigger than the problem.

5) Self-Capitalization
We're now ready to talk about *capitalizing* on yourself on your mind-emotions, talents, skills, and circumstances. That means finding your passion and talents. It means synergizing your passions with your talents, turn them into skills, and then externalizing the internal richness that results as you play to our strengths. In this, *being* wealth comes before *doing* wealth and *having* wealth. Wealth is first an internal creation, a mind that creates values and solves problems that enriches the lives of others.

Who do you need to become so that you can fully capitalize on your mind, body, emotions, talents, and dispositions? Have you developed a self-evaluation and self-esteeming that allows you to stay resiliently resourceful during the times of uncertainty? This is the foundation for decisiveness, the ability to quickly make up your mind when facing an opportunity. How are you currently capitalizing on your strengths? What will be the next thing you will do to capitalize on your creativity? How can you create multiple streams of income from the same passion?

6) Self-Optimism[2]
What does it take to have a basic and core optimism about yourself as a human being? We know that wealth creation generally requires an optimism in what you can do and the value you can add. Yet it requires more. It requires an even more core optimism about life itself and especially about the unpleasant things that happen. And while it requires being able to *see* opportunities and proactively *seize* the opportunities that fit for your singularity, it involves something even more fundamental.

Basic optimism is an attitude of excellence that enables you to stay motivated, determined, open, creative, persevering and resilient especially in the face of difficulties and hard times. When you bring *optimism* to your wealth creation, you are empowered to *see* things with a sense of delight, joy, pleasantness, motivation, warmth, etc. It just makes things go a lot better than to approach things with any other attitude.

The deeper and more core optimism is one about yourself, others, and life. This is an optimism that can keep hurt and evil out so that it does not darken your inner world and make you a pessimist about human nature or life. To understand this we need to understand the structure of optimism and its opposite, learned helplessness. This comes from the research work of Martin Seligman (1975, 1990) on "learned helplessness" and "learned optimism."

Learned helplessness refers to a contamination of a person's mind and heart with a pessimism and skepticism so that a person frames a "negative" event when something "bad" happens. When a person does this, it creates a particular *explanatory style* for self, others, and life. When that happens, a person then interprets most things in a way that contaminates them and undermines their ability to move forward. Seligman defines the learned helpleness explanatory style in these three terms:

- *The source of the evil and hurt is* **Personal.** You interpret the problem as you—you are the problem. Your inner self is inadequate, flawed, or problematic.
- *The time element then becomes* **Permanent**. You interpret the hurt or evil as unchangeable, insoluble, and insurmountable. It is permanent. Forever.
- *The space wherein this occurs is* **Pervasive.** You see it as everywhere. You see it as effecting everything and undermining every facet of your life.

Together these three **P**s of personal, permanent, and pervasive create the gestalt of "pessimism" so that the person with learned helplessness (as the opposite of core optimism) sees him or herself as inadequate and deficient, as lacking the means, ability, and motivation to do anything about it, to make a difference in life, to improve the quality of life.

So how can you create a de-contamination of this horrendous state and create an optimism to replace the pessimism? To create a core optimism requires that you keep the hurt or evil out from your central or core self. How do you do that? This optimistic explanatory style does it by

framing hurtful events in a way that allows you to stay optimistic about yourself, others, human nature, and life itself. It does so with three opposite perspectives:
- *The source of the hurt or evil is* **External.**   Now you interpret the problem as about some event, thing, or situation out there, not about you.
- *The time of the hurt is* **Temporary.** It is about this particular person or situation, and it is not forever. Now you interpret the problem as here ... now ... and you keep it there in your perspective.
- *The space of the hurt is* **Specific.**   It is in this moment; it is in this space about this thing. Now you interpret the problem as not about everything, just this one thing.

To create the core optimism state for yourself, you can use the three *nots*— not me, not forever, not everywhere as an antidote for the deep pessimism that comes from the three Ps. With this formulation, you can now utter the three magical words about a painful or distressing event that took the spirit out of you, the event that you experiences as a hurt or an evil. If it was in the past, then you can say: *"That Then There!"* Or if it is current, the you can say: *"This here now!"*

What if you don't have a core optimism within you because some old past hurt has contaminated you, your spirit, your attitude, and your basic orientation in the world. What then?

First, identify the reference situation that is calling for optimism from you. When or where in the process of taking action to create wealth do you most need optimism?

Next, identify the situation in which you might be tempted to become pessimistic. What is that situation? What is the triggering situation? When and where are you typically blind to opportunities? What comes to mind? Is there a reference experience?

Once you have that, then hold that referent event in mind, and meta-state yourself with the anti-Ps of pessimism. To do this, you'll want to access the three *not*-states and use them to push out the old distortions. First access the state of *"Not-Me!"* Feel it, and gesture it in response to the trigger. Then bring "Not everywhere" and *"not* forever" states to your primary state. In its place put, "This event, this day."

Now test it. How much have you pushed it away? How much more do you need to push it away? Keep doing this until you have the feeling that you have pushed out from you the idea and the feeling that the bad thing was "me," "everywhere" and "forever."

Test it again for de-contamination. Are you de-contaminated from the pessimism and skepticism? Is there any more of the old referent event influencing you and your interpretative style? As you test your state, what is there? If you have pushed the learned helplessness interpretative style out, it should leave you now able to recover a child-like optimism. Does it? This will be the cue that you have succeeded.

Playfully experiment with bringing other resourceful states. Here are some possible resources to use:
- *Possibility:* It's possible to achieve something.
- *Desirability:* It's desirable to aim for, work toward, and invest time, energy, money, etc. into making a difference.
- *Resources:* There are abundant resources available; I can even bring abundant resources that don't now exist into existence.
- *Self-Worth:* My worth and value is a given.
- *Significance:* It's worth doing, valuable, and we have the esteem, value, significance that makes us worthy and deserving to do it.
- *Playful:* Humor lightens things and enables me to be real as it also facilitates greater creativity.
- *Passion:* Loving what I do and the difference I make keeps me focused on what really matters.
- *Vision:* Seeing the dream that excites me and casts light on my path.

Continue until the gestalt state of optimism emerges. Does this yet generate the perspective, frame of mind, or state of optimism? What else needs to be added? Have you added each resource sufficiently? Now put it into your future. As you now imagine moving through life with this attitude in the weeks and months to come, how does that settle? Are you aligned with this? Any objections? Do you want to keep this? How will you?

7) Self-Investment
The next development of self for wealth creation is self-investment. There's a reason for this—you create wealth by investing in your

ongoing development. Blotnick spoke about this in these words:

> "People who didn't become rich tended to think in Stage 2 ways— first I'll make my money, then I'll read, write, do musicals, travel, etc. They didn't think about *investing in themselves.*" (p. 94)
>
> "To put it bluntly, if you only have $100,000 or less to invest, there is *no* place you can reasonably invest it ... except in yourself." (p. 95)
>
> "What characterized those who eventually became rich was their willingness to spend time and money pursuing on their own any aspect of their work they found fascinating." (p. 244)

There's many ways to do this, here are a number of them for your consideration:

a) Develop your mind as your source of wealth.
As opportunities are not seen with physical eyes but with the eye of your mind, you have to train your mind in creativity, practical knowledge, curiosity, etc. And since wealth is created by solving problems, develop your critical thinking skills.

b) Become a life-long learner.
While self-investment takes many different forms, at its heart it means becoming a life-long learner. Wealth inherently lies in the ability to learn—to learn effectively and to accelerate the learning so that you learn faster than your competition. This will become even more true as business moves increasingly more into the information age. So, are you continuously reading, learning, and adding to your knowledge base?

> *The best investment you'll ever make is investing in yourself:*
>
> "To put it bluntly, if you only have $100,000 or less to invest, there is *no* place you can reasonably invest it ... except in yourself."
>   Scrully Blotnick

For the pro, school is never out. You are forever learning new answers, new questions, new possibilities. Plan for life-long learning. Get a steady diet of exposing yourself to new information every day. This feeds your ability to see opportunities.

Stephen Arterburn speaks about the learning mode as the key that will enable you to become a collector of wisdom. He comments that he doesn't know anyone in business who is successful and who doesn't read

a lot. He then suggests that you ask:
> "How can I use this knowledge given my chosen vocation? What concepts in this course can I leverage in helping make my operation more productive?"

Donald Trump:
> "Money may not grow from trees, but it does grow from talent, hard work, and brains." (47). My financial IQ is constantly improving as I watch over my many businesses and my staff. Good investors are good students." (2004, p. 49)

Robert Kiyosaki:
> "Your most single powerful asset—your mind. An untrained mind creates poverty." (p. 104)

Ebony asked prominent black achievers to speak in the series, "If I were Young Again." Paul R. Williams, famous architect said:
> "Whatever one does as a profession or livelihood, he should endeavor to read the current magazines pertaining to his work. One must keep pace with progress and what the other fellow is thinking and doing. In order to do this he must read–read–read!!! He should strive to become a specialist and not just *another* architect, engineer, or salesman." (*Ebony,* 18:10, August, 1963, p. 56)

Napoleon Hill
> "Successful men in all callings never stop acquiring specialized knowledge related to their major purpose, business, or profession. Those who are not successful usually make the mistake of believing that the knowledge-acquiring period ends when one finishes school." (p. 79).

c) Seek continuous improvement.
The kaizen principle of continuous improvement means that after you learn a new skill, you don't stop learning about that skill or how to use it. But you'll continue to discover how to keep improving. The goal I set several years ago is to improve 5% a year as a writer, as a trainer, and as a coach. It means continually using the power of incremental improvement. What about you?

d) Develop your creativity.
Self-Actualization Psychology recognizes that human nature is innately creative. Creativity is our heritage as human beings. We are always

putting things together to create new forms. We are always associating things in new combinations. Creativity is thinking out of the box; it is willing to be unique and different, it is experimenting, it is playing with ideas and words.

> "What do most millionaires tell me they learned? ... they learned to *think differently from the crowd.*" (Stanley, 2000, p. 22)
> "Questioning the norm, the status quo, and authority are hallmarks of the thinking of self-made millionaires and those destined to become affluent." (92)

Blotnick:
> "In allowing themselves to try a variety of different approaches to their field, they finally hit upon the one which worked best for them. They weren't necessarily more ambitious, smarter, or more talented. They gave themselves the opportunity to locate what for them was the right angle of attack..." (p. 92)

Your creativity will enable you to refuse to accept the restrictions of your job. When you have a job, you are paid to *not* do other things. Yet by becoming creative you can discover ways to follow your passion anyway and new ways to create value.

e) Develop the flexibility of expanding your choices and responses.
Millionaires condition their minds to offset fears through mental toughness. They develop an attitude of love for their products and services. *Flexibility* is part of creativity: experimenting, exploring new things. Peter Drucker writes:

> "We now know that the source of wealth is something specifically human: *knowledge.* If we apply knowledge to tasks we already know how to do, we call it 'productivity.' If we apply knowledge to tasks that are new and different, we call it 'innovation.' Only knowledge allows us to achieve these goals." (*Managing for Future,* p. 24, 1992)

The Mental Wealth Principle:
Wealth is a state of mind and is developed through the wealth of a rich creative mind.

f) Refuse to let schooling and degrees to stop you.
If wealth is built as you invest in your minds and your creativity, then don't let school or formal schooling get in the way of your mind and

education. Distinguish your schooling from your education. After all, a lot of "schooling" isn't education anyway. True education draws out what's within you (that's what the word means.) Jim Rohn writes:

> "With formal education you can earn a living, with self education, you can earn a fortune."

g) Learn to think like a millionaire.
Thomas Stanley (2000) wrote that the self-made millionaires of his study are "... proficient at controlling their thought processes." They were able to use their thinking processes so they would act in ways that would lead to success.

> "The reason that so few people are financially independent today is that they place many negative roadblocks in their heads. *Becoming wealthy is, in fact, a mind game.* ... Before you can become a millionaire, you must *learn to think like one.* You must learn how to motivate yourself constantly to counter fear with courage." (135)

h) Swim against the current.
> "It's unfortunate that most non-millionaires accept the negative evaluations given them by authority figures. ... the millionaires had the insight, courage, and audacity to challenge the assessments made by teachers, professors, amateur critics, and the Educational Testing Service." (101).

8) Self-Integrity

Integrity is saying what you will do and *doing* what you say. Integrity, as a strong and steadfast adherence to your principles, requires a strong sense of yourself and your value, enabling you to be undivided in your passions. This generates the gestalt

> **The Integrity Principle:**
> *Wealth is built by the integrity which gives us the character and power of congruency.*

of a larger sense of wholeness and soundness in mind and body.

How do millionaires think that differs from non-millionaires? Stanley (2000) found that they frequently think and examine themselves in terms of their self-integrity. They focus on such things as being honest with all people (integrity), applying self-control (discipline), getting along with people (social skills), having a supportive spouse, and working harder than most people (p. 11). When these facets come together, we call them *character*. Stanley and Danko write:

> "What kind of businesses do millionaires own? All kinds. You can't predict if someone is a millionaire by the type of business. After 20 years of studying millionaires, we have concluded that *the character of the business owner* is more important in predicting his level of wealth than the classification of his business." (p. 228)

The benefits of integrity are many. There is the peace of mind that comes when you know you are doing your best. There is the security of congruency as you know that you are aligned with your highest beliefs and values. Then you can rest in your actions knowing that they are sufficient and that you never have to worry about the past catching up and finding you out. There is also the sense of being stable in yourself. Thomas Stanley (2000) speak of this stability:

> "Without the conditioning to be stable, it's an uphill climb to become an economic success. Conversely, the unstable tend to be unfocused and temperamental, and they have difficulty getting along with people, including their spouses and their children. They also tend to lack the determination and resolve to deal with recurring economic threats, risks, fears, and worries." (p. 172)

How to develop Integrity:
a) Be mindful of what you say.
Clarify for yourself your own understandings about your values and beliefs that you want to play a significant role in your wealth creation plan. As you come to know yourself more intimately— what's really important to you and how you work best, you'll be able to communicate more clearly to others. Aim to be increasingly more mindful of your communications—what you say, what you don't say, what you promise, etc. *Treat your word as a sacred trust.* Don't give it mindlessly. Stop your "gift of gab" if you are quick to speak.

b) Do what you say you will do.
Your sense of self and congruence are more important than all of your public image skills. Knowing and acting on your values and your purpose gives you congruence. And being congruent with your values gives you personal power to make you trustworthy in the eyes of others. Do what you say you will do. If your words are a sacred trust to others, then go out of your way to fulfill them. If you can't fulfill your word, let the people impacted know that. Then apologize and make it as right as you can.

c) Make yourself accountable to someone.
Who will you appoint to hold you accountable? The way to develop a good relationship with yourself and what you say, promise, and do is to have an accountability structure. As a state of alignment, congruence arises when you believe in what you are doing and your body and mind are working towards your goal.

d) Look for feedback.
Keep an eye on your actions in order to develop a consistency of your actions with your words.

> Stop trying to balance work and play. Instead make your work more pleasurable. For millionaires, work and pleasure are one and the same. I'm always looking for ideas and inspiration that I can adopt. Create an integrated lifestyle. Aim for integration rather than balance.
> Donald Trump

Wealth's Dimensions

Throughout these pages, I have been referring to the three dimensions of wealth— *being, doing,* and *having*. Robert Kiyosaki also speaks of these three dimensions. He says that it is first *who* you have to *be* that counts—your beliefs and attitudes. If you are a person with a loser mentality, you will always lose. That's why self-development comes first. First become *rich* inside yourself— in your identity, self-definition. Then eternalize that inner wealth.

- *Being:* The wealth of *being* is your internal experience—it is your wealth of thoughts, ideas, and emotions that inspire you for new and creative ways to add value to others.
- *Doing:* What do you actually *do* to create value and abundance in the world. This is the wealth of your energy, speech, skills, abilities, etc. It could also be the wealth of models, plans, inventions, procedures, etc. that you create that gives more value to people.
- *Having:* The wealth of *having* results from *being* and *doing*. This is the wealth that you enjoy from your work and commitment.

The Inside-Out Wealth Pattern

The heart and core of wealth is a rich mind and heart full of ideas that can solve problems and a rich set of skills that can make this real in the world. Wealth is not money, it is adding value that increases the quality of life. In developing your wealth engine, first develop your own inner wealth.

First, access a sense of "value" and valuing. Do this by taking a moment to consider, What do you value? What do you appreciate as valuable and precious? Is there anything really, really important to you? What? What evokes a strong sense of the value of something? As you think of that and experience the feelings of valuing ... what's that like? What else allows you to experience *valuing*? As you recall these, keep amplifying this state until it is a 9 on a scale of 0 to 10.

Apply this state of valuing to yourself. As you feel this state about yourself, and apply to self, what does it feel like when the gestalt of self-value, self-worth, self-esteem emerges? "I'm important!" "I count!" "I deserve to have the good things of life like everybody else." "I am a learner, creative, flexible, operating from abundance, and have integrity."

Apply to your powers of response. Notice what happens when you apply this to your thoughts-feelings and speech and behavior. What gestalts emerge when you do this? Let it emerge as an appreciation of your talents and skills, "I can contribute! I have much to contribute." Notice your sense of creativity, that you have a rich mind-heart system, that there's abundance. "I create wealth through courage, persistence, resilience, efficiency, and fun."

Apply this valuing state to your work and the whole of life. Scan your world of work with *valuing* in mind and notice how that transforms things. Install these words:
> "How can I add value here? If this was my business, what could I do that might make it more valuable to the customers, to my fellow employees, to my boss, etc.? What problems can I find and how can I bring my internal richness of mind-and-emotion to find solutions?"

Add sufficient supporting frames. What belief would support this? What intention, decision, metaphor, understanding, etc. would support this? Add in belief frames about abundance, creativity, opportunity.

Future pace and quality control. As you imagine taking this into the days and weeks to come, are all parts of your mind-body system aligned with this? Do you like this? Are you ready to do this? Are you really to allow this to increasingly become your operational program in the future?

Commission with your executive frame of mind. Will the executive part of your mind take responsibility to make this yours?

My Personal Story
Sometime after I recognized myself as a wealth creator, I took that on as part of my identity. I then found myself facing some new and fascinating questions.

> "What wealth am I creating today?" "How can I create more opportunities for others to create wealth?" "How will this project, research, or training create wealth for people?"

I also often sensed that the unleashing of actualizing processes that I present will increase their income. Sometimes I get feedback that reveals that their income doubled, tripled, and even quadrupled after a coaching session or a training. And today, when that happens, I always take a moment to feel the pleasure, "I am a Wealth Creator."

While these were new questions for me, I welcomed them because they created a new orientation for me. And with them I began creating training manuals and programs that would not end just with myself, but that I made available for others. They are now known as the Gateway trainings of Neuro-Semantics and are offered by scores of trainers around the world. And with each new program or book or pattern, I reinforce my identity as a wealth creator.

Your Adventure in Creating Wealth
As your Wealth Coach, this chapter offers you some powerful leveraging activities. Are you ready to become a Wealth Creator in your identity? Are your ready to make as many people wealthy as you can? If so, are there any interferences that you might need to deal with, anything preventing you from taking on the identity and role of being a wealth creator?

Grab your *Wealth Creative Adventure Journal* and make a list of any and every interference to your Wealth Creator identity. As you step back, what are the beliefs, understandings, or decisions that create this interference? Now scan through this chapter again looking for more empowering beliefs and meanings.

> Do you need to use the Meta-Yes pattern again for installing some enhancing beliefs about yourself as a Wealth Creator?

How well have you made the distinction between yourself as a human being and as a human doer? How much more clear and definitive do you need to make that distinction so that you don't "have to prove anything?" If you're having any challenge with this, make a list of all the reasons why distinguishing self-esteem from self-confidence will free you to create wealth.

How solidly do you have an inner sense of self-optimism? What do you need to do to completely eliminate the three **P**s (personal, permanent, pervasive) that make up learned helplessness. Then you can replace it with the three **T**s (that, there, then) that keeps you from bringing in a hurt and contaminating your inner self. This creates learned optimism at your core.

As you now consider creating being a Wealth Creator as part of your new identity, have you made that decision? Will you? Is that who you are or are becoming? Do you see yourself as a wealth creator? What would it take to identify yourself as a wealth creator?

Also make sure you have clearly *set the person / behavior distinction* in your mind. Have you fully separated yourself as a person from what you do? What do you need to do to set that distinction in yourself? Once you do that, then set the frame of *being* as a human being so you can then *do*. Meta-state your sense of self as a human being with acceptance and esteem. Meta-state your sense of self as an achiever with appreciation of what you can do and contribute.[3]

End of Chapter Notes:

1. The central pattern for developing a robust sense of self is the self-acceptance, self-appreciation, and self-esteem pattern that is in the APG workshop. You can find this also in *Secrets of Personal Mastery* (1997).

2. See *Meta-States* chapters on Resilience (chapters 4 and 5).

3. The process of meta-stating is a process of bringing one state to a previous state in such a way that you put the new state in a meta (or higher) position. As such, the meta-state then sets the frame or context for the previous state. If you bring joy and delight to learning, then *joyful* becomes the higher state and frames the previous state of *learning*. The result is a meta-state of *joyful learning*.

Chapter 9

WHO WILL GO WITH ME?

*"If you want to be rich in the truest sense of the word,
it can't only be about you.
It has to include adding value to other people's lives."*
Harv Eker

*"Money is a measure of the value that people pay
for goods and services. The amount of money you earn
is the measure of the value that others place on your contribution."*
Brian Tracy

Ultimately business success, wealth creation, leadership and management, are all about relationships. In all of these domains, it is all about working *with* and *through* people. And regarding wealth, no one creates wealth alone or becomes rich by him or herself. *Creating wealth is always a relational event.*

Is that shocking? Does that surprise you? Given that this is what the research consistently reveals, then consider these questions for your own wealth creation:

- How are you going to receive money if not from people who want what you have to offer?
- Who wants what you have to offer?
- How are you going to create the product, service, or experience by yourself? Will you need no one to supply anything for you to

make that happen?
- Who will you need as customers, suppliers, marketing and sales people, supporters, shareholders, colleagues, etc.?

Even Bill Gates, who for many years has been on the richest men in America, did not do it alone. He did it with valued colleagues. For years, the second richest man in America was Paul Allen, his vice president. In fact, several of his vice-presidents have been on the list of the richest people in the US. In other words, *as* he became wealthy, so did many others. He brought many others along with him in the process, or perhaps we could say, *they did it together.* And this is an important principle in wealth creation—we create with others and through others. *Creating wealth is a team process,* it involves a community of people.

The People Principle: *Wealth is created as you work with and through people. This necessitates clear and compelling communication for understanding, rapport, and negotiations.*

To extend on the previous chapter, this means that you not only become a wealth creator in yourself, but we become a group of *collaborative* wealth creators. That's because of the collaborative wealth principle of the relational dimension of wealth creation—wealth creation is a collaborative event. And if it is a collaborative event, it involves several key collaborations:
- Communicating effectively in a way that aligns and inspires everybody involved.
- Creating win/win collaborative arrangements so that we experience of synergy in the interpersonal interactions.
- Networking with others to create collaborative partnerships that continuously opens up new possibilities.
- Speaking the truth honestly with each other to be authentically open.

Beyond Competitiveness

If *inside-out wealth* involves being collaborative and cooperative, then what is the role of competitiveness? How useful or un-useful is the competitive spirit in business?

At first glance, it seems that you need to be competitive in order to create wealth and succeed in business. And this does seem to be true at the first levels. When you begin, you need to have enough "aggressiveness" to know and go for what you want. Aggressiveness, in this sense, simply refers to *going at* (aggressing) or toward what you want. It is not about being angry. It is about being determined and committed so that you take action, you initiate possibilities, and you take informed risks similar to a competitor in a sports event seeking to be faster, stronger, or more skilled than his or her competitors. Healthy competitiveness is not about putting someone down or gaining unfair advantage over others. It is about developing to your highest and best skills and potentials that challenges others to do better.

It is at the beginning also that pitting your skills and energies against others can get you moving and create an excitement that keeps you motivated. Typically, having someone or something to beat mobilizes energies. Top athletes know this. They look for a good competitor, someone close, or even better than they are, so that they are put to the test and push forward to new levels of excellence. That's why world records are most often broken when a whole group of top athletes are competing. This kind of respectful and collegial cooperation makes it a powerful force driving toward peak performance. When the competition itself is respectful and honorable it entails good sportsmanship and good attitude. The best competition occurs within a context of collaboration. So as a meta-state, it is *collaborative* competition.

Competition can, and often does, become sick and toxic. This happens when competition becomes disrespectful and malicious. When people compete without respect for their competitors, without appreciation for the value that a good competitor offers, and without an honorable sense of fairness, then competition turns toxic. That's when competitors become unethical and do underhanded things to gain unfair advantage. Then competition becomes vicious, cruel, and inhumane.

The mere fact that you are seeking to compete against another, or against a standard or record, does not in itself conflict with collaborating. In fact, it takes a healthy state of respect and honor to collaborate enough so that the competitive can be useful in pushing you and others forward so everyone gives their best efforts. Competing can add fun, zest, and excitement *if it arises from an attitude of respect and fair play.* Without that, it degenerates into ugly attitudes and hurtful behaviors.

Blotnick's 1960 to 1980 longitudinal research into those who became millionaires demonstrated several things about competitiveness:

>First, the competitiveness of those who were highly competitive backfired badly as the years passed. It became increasingly destructive and so undermined their long-term success in becoming rich.
>
>Second, the competitor's nightmare is "avoiding a loss." This fear drives them to compete and simultaneously prevents them from collaborating.
>
>Third, competitive creates a small-minded local focus suggesting that the person's ego is in the way which prevents healthy cooperation.
>
>Fourth, those who became rich became less and less competitive as they rose to the top. After all, companies and employers require team spirit. They want, and require, that their top people to foster a spirit of cooperation.

What's needed then is a collaborative attitude or frame of mind so that you look at others as possible collaborators and partners. Do you have that? Or do you naturally default to distrusting people and being paranoid about what they are doing and what they are trying to steal from you? Do you interpret the excellence and success of another as somehow taking something away from you? Do you put your personal value (self-esteem) on the line by always comparing your success against that of others? How easily do you fall into complaints about others or end up playing the Blame Game?

All of this identifies the importance of trust over distrust in being a wealth creator. And, to build trust you have to be trustworthy. That is, you have to be true and loyal in order to build loyalty in others. And to do that with others raises the assumptive beliefs you have about people. Are people, in their core nature, trustworthy or untrustworthy? What do you believe about human nature? This is the question that separates people who operate from Theory X in business and Theory Y of management.[1]

>**The Collaboration Principle:**
>Wealth is created through cooperating with others, networking, finding mentors, being mentors, and other ways to collaborate.

Who will go with you? If you can't do it alone and if you have to build collaborative partnerships, *how* do you do that? What are the relational skills that you'll need to develop and apply as you become a collaborative wealth creator?

    1) Trustworthy. Become trustworthy in yourself in order to attract trustworthy people to you and to create a culture of trust.

    2) Open Communication. Communicate openly and forthrightly without secrets or hidden agendas.

    3) Open Confrontation. Deal with issues and problems when they are small and manageable.

    4) Supportive Communication. Communicate and relate in ways that are supportive of others.

    5) Team Spirit. Focus on building a team spirit with others, a sense of "we" are in this together.

    6) Negotiate for win/win arrangements. Create agreements that allows everyone to win and refuse any that are one-sided.

    7) Defuse others. When people reach limits of their stress, move into defusing.

    8) Modeling. Find best practices and examples of excellence and model the structure of that experience.

    9) Networking. Keep open your possibilities for finding and connecting with potential collaborative partners.

In this, wealth creation is inevitably grounded in effective relational and social skills. This means you will need to be able to make accurate judgments about people, "read" them in terms of their values and response style, gain rapport, create win/win arrangements, collaborate, work together, etc.

1) Trustworthy
It all begins with trust. You can't really do business with anyone if you don't trust them or if they don't trust you. And that means that people can trust your word, trust that what you say you will do, trust that what you describe is true to the best of your knowledge, trust that you will not harm, deceive, or cheat them, trust that you will be the person you present yourself to be, and trust that your promises are good as gold.

Are you that trustworthy? *Being worthy of the trust of others* means you have the character that people can depend on. Without trust, business breaks down because relationship breaks down because communication breaks down. When that happens then about the only way to proceed is by rules and laws. And when people won't be held accountable by rules and laws, so does all business between the individuals.

Do people trust you? Do they know that you will be as good as your word? That your word and handshake are as solid as a signed contract? Can they depend on you to arrive when you say you will? That you'll complete a project when you say you will? And that if something comes up, you will let them know and keep them informed? These are a few of the ways that we build trust and become trustworthy in the eyes of others.

In business and in the process of collaboratively creating wealth with others, can people trust that you will actively listen, care about their view and opinion, clarify data while communicating, say what is true and correct yourself when you make a mistake? Can they trust that you will do that? That you will reach out to connect, to create rapport with them, and to be receptive to them? If they can, then it will be easy for you to find and attract the kind of people that you can build a successful, productive, and profitable business with.[2]

2) Open Communication
While almost all communication with people always needs to be open communication, this is especially important for successful businesses. The reason should be obvious, you need to let others know what you are doing and why, what you want and why, what others can expect from you, and have an openness to keep checking out your communications so that you're on the same page.

How you communicate determines how you relate and how you relate governs how you communicate. Actually both of these words describe the same thing—the way you talk and act with others. And so *communication* actually involves everything that goes into how you treat others. Constantly being late for appointments is a communication. Judging and criticizing and never acknowledging what someone is doing well is also a communication.[3]

Open communicating and relating is critical so that you know who you are working with and what you can expect. When expectations are constantly violated, you feel that you don't know the other person and don't know what to anticipate. Open communication contrasts with keeping secrets or distrusting others and only giving them as much information as *you* think they need to know. Research about great companies and effective leaders today support the importance of open communication and getting beyond the paranoia of playing your hand close to your chest. And for more about open book management as well as open communication practices, see *Unleashing Leadership*.

There are a great many communication skills that support wealth creation. They involve asking, exploring, leveling, negotiating, selling, influencing, encouraging, inspiring, planning, brainstorming, etc. The most fundamental communication skill is the ability to simply ask for what you want and to do so in a forthright way. This is the foundation for the ability to negotiate from a win/win orientation.

This is where many entrepreneurs, business owners, and leaders fail. They create processes that eventually prevent "bad news" from reaching them. They do not receive feedback because any conflictual or "negative" information is filtered out long before it gets to them.

3) Open Confrontation

Confrontation? Really? While it may seem contradictory to good communication, actually the best communication and the most open communication between people is the communication skills that allow you to "confront" each other and deal with issues when they are small and manageable and not wait until they are large and unmanageable.

Open confrontation isn't about being mean or harsh or "in your face" with another person. It means having the openness to bring up what otherwise might be sensitive about a "touchy" subjects. It refers to simply putting it on the table so you can talk about it. When done with a caring tone of voice and attitude, confronting each other helps to keep things current and address differences in a healthy and respectful way.

The irony is that *conflict* is more often than not a positive experience for growth, deeper understanding, encountering oneself, changing, and finding new arenas for adding value. Conflict is natural and provides an organic process for clearing out the things that undermine a person's success. And yet, most people and most companies are conflict avoidant. We create styles of communicating and relating to eliminate facing up to the conflicts that could become highly useful.[4]

4) Supportive Communication

If open communication focuses on clarity, precision, and forthrightness, then supportive communication focuses on connecting, building rapport, safety, and adding the personal touch. Communication that supports more flexibly adjusts to the hearer and takes time to consider the listener's style for processing information and communicating. This dimension of communication recognizes that it is not just the exchange of data and transfer of information, it is also the emotions, feelings, and states that each person brings to the communicating.

Because you communicate from state to state, from your state to the state of the other person, in supportive communication you consciously aim to elicit the kind of states in others that enables them to hear more effectively and respond positively. This requires the awareness of the state that both are in and the ability to elicit states.

The process of wealth creating requires the ability to support others and to be supported. When you operate from a win/win attitude, it's easy to be supportive of others, to be able to celebrate in their success, to experience empathy (take second position to another) with them and for them. And it is this attitude that moves a person away from the scarcity thinking that feeds competition, greed, grabbing, putting others down to feel higher, etc.

5) Team Spirit

In Blotnick's study those who succeeded in becoming wealthy also became increasingly non-competitive in their attitude over time. The longer they stayed with their passion, they less competitive they became with their co-workers. They became more cooperative as they adopted more of a win/win attitude.

As you become more of a collaborator, you will naturally be thinking about building your own personal wealth creation team. Are you willing to find and create a support group to keep yourself on track with your wealth creation plan?
- Do you have a team? Whose on your team?
- Who are your key business partners?
- Who else do you need on your team?
- How is your relationship with your suppliers?
- Manufactures?
- Customers and clients?

- Sales people?

Having colleagues gives you the chance of letting others hold you accountable to your goals and plans. Whether it will be one person or many, what's your plan for accountability?
- Who can I appoint to hold me responsible to my goals?
- Who will I give permission to ask me accountability questions so that I can stay on target?
- Who can you share your weekly, monthly, and yearly goals?
- Have you updated your wealth creation plan this month?
- What have you done today to act on your plan?
- What other ideas do you have for putting this idea into action?

Once you have one or more persons who will hold you accountable, then you can have that person call you once a week with a set of pre-designed questions something like the following. Originally I created this list for myself and gave it to the people I appointed to hold me accountable to my wealth creation plan:
- How are you doing this week?
- How did you do this week on keeping to your budget?
- How well did you control your spending?
- Did you practice frugality this week? How did you do that?
- What will you be doing next week to increase your best states for creating wealth?
- Did you save 10% this last week?
- How did you work on becoming richer inside?
- What action plans are you working on today?

With people on your team, you have people with whom you can engage in brainstorming that will increase your brain power. That's because there is synergy when mind acts upon mind in a context of acceptance, playfulness, exploration, curiosity, etc.

Criteria for Deciding With Whom to Work

How do you decide on people to work with? How do you choose an accountant, attorney, or other professional people with whom to work? It depends on your best work style and your values. So obviously, the more

> **Negotiation Principles:**
> Wealth is created by negotiating win/win deals. Your power to negotiate is your ability to add value to others.

clear you are about yourself, the more you can communicate that to others. That allows both you and the other to make a clear decision about whether there is a fit or not. My criteria for my decisions include the following. Feel free to use and adapt the following for your own situation.

Criteria for Choosing others who fit with my Style:
1) An openness for conversation and questions.

>A big part of my style is that I want to learn as I work. So I like asking lots of questions and talking through things to make sure that I am on the same page with the person. So when I first meet a new person, I will ask lots of questions and watch how the person responds. "Will the person support my learning or does he find it an irritant and something to endure?"

2) A quick responsiveness for exchanging information.

>I want to know about the person's responsiveness. Is the person responsive? How long does it take the person to respond to calls, emails, etc. My basic style is to respond to all calls and emails within 24 hours. And that's what I prefer in the people I work with. If that is too intense or demanding, then I will continue to look for someone who shares those values.

3) A collaborative style.

>Is the person collaborative in style? Or does the person seem to play games? Does the person use manipulative language patterns? My style is collaborative, open, and forthright. Since I operate from the idea of abundance, that's what I want from others. If a person operates from scarcity, watching his or her back, suspiciousness, distrust, etc., I just don't want to be a part of that. It does not fit for me.

4) An openness in terms of information sharing.

>Does the person openly provide information or is he or she secretive? How does the person provide information? For example, I have a mortgage leader who puts out a monthly newsletter that I look forward to. In it he puts critical information about changes in laws, taxes, etc. and recommendations. Does the person take the initiative to share or do I have to pull the information out of him or her?

5) A sense of fun and enjoyment.
>Do I enjoy the person? Does laughter naturally occur, or is everything "strictly business?" Do we share a similar humor? Is the humor respectful?

6) An openness to conflict resolution skills.
>How does the person work through a conflict? Talk it out? Yell? Will the person stay engaged or give up and avoid? My style is direct, forthright, and confrontational; I want to deal with things when they are small and manageable and ideally to talk things out to a win/win solution. To achieve that, raising the voice is fine as far as I'm concerned as long as we can stay focused on the issue and be respectful. I know how to defuse and I appreciate that in others. Does the person live in the past and keep resentments?

7) Open to feedback.
>Is the person open to feedback? Does the person seek it and ask for feedback or is the person avoidant of feedback, overly sensitive to it, and defensive?

6) Negotiating

If wealth is a collaborative process, then you'll need the ability to negotiate effectively with people. Wealth is created by negotiating and negotiating arrangements wherein everybody wins. Win/win arrangements enables everyone to feel good about the deals that we co-create. Your power to negotiate is your ability to add value to others and to the project you are engaged in.

What do you believe? Do you believe that everything is negotiable? Do you believe that you can almost always create great win/win negotiations? What beliefs will you need to release and dismiss in order to negotiate in effective and respectful ways? There is an art to creating win/win negotiations with others. To learn that art requires some particular beliefs and communication skills.

1) Openly identify what each person wants.
>What do you want? What do I want?
>Why do I want that? What will it give me?
>Why do you want that? What will it give you?
>How do you know that I want this?

What other ways could each of us obtain what we want?

2) Access your best state for communicating a negotiation.
What is the best state you need to be in to start the communications? The menu list might include: caring, pleasant, relaxed, harmony, empathetic, listening, excited, etc. What do you need?
Do you know how to access that state?
How easily can you do that?

3) Take time to understand the other person or persons.
What does the other person or persons want?
Do you know how to inquire to discover?
Are you willing to ask outcome questions and listen with a third-ear for the other's wants, values, dis-values, meanings, emotions, thinking patterns, etc.?

4) Engage in an appreciative dialogue to co-create a workable arrangement.
Is there a fittingness between us?
Can we co-create a win/win relationship?
What will it take?
What will we each obtain from this?
What else could we create?
What questions have we not asked that might create even something more valuable?

5) Identify the range of your positions.
What are the boundaries of your goals and outcomes?
Do you know what's acceptable, what is your ideal outcome, what is not acceptable?
How much flexibility do you have?
What could increase your flexibility?
What other values can you give?

7) Defusing

Another wealth creation collaborative skill is one that you probably would not include on your first list. Yet *defusing* is exactly that. The skill and art of defusing someone who is upset, angry, scared, stressed-out, or in a cranky mood is a true gift to another human being. Now true enough, we typically do not think of it as a gift; typically it feels hard and conflictual.

Yet in all endeavors where human beings are involved there is going to be emotions and sometimes unpleasant emotions. In fact, most people experience what we call the "negative" emotions as unpleasant and stressful: anger, fear, sadness, grief, frustration, disappointment, upset, shocked, shame, guilt, etc. And when we experience these emotions, typically our stress level goes up. Our state changes.

If continued, we get into a high stress state and then at a certain point we enter into the fight-flight-freeze stage. That's when a qualitative change occurs. At a certain point, our higher cortex, consciously or unconsciously, cues one of two messages, either "Danger!" or "Overload!" In either case, blood is then withdraw from brain and stomach and sent to the larger muscle groups for fighting, fleeing, or freezing. And with that we go into either-or thinking and so we are literally and physically not able to think as clearly as we otherwise could.

Now the moment has come for defusing. Defusing is the skill of helping a person defuse, unload, and release the stresses and negative feelings—to say words and talk out the stress rather than act it out. Of course the trick for the defuser is to understand what's happening. When you can do that, then you can also empathize with the person, enable the person to feel understood and safe, and stop yourself from doing anything else. It is *not* time for business communication, negotiating, or any other talk. It is only time for the other person to talk through the stressful thoughts and release the negative emotions.

If you can do that for another. or if someone can do that for you, the relationship is protected. The person is helped from unnecessary fighting or fleeing, a fight is averted, and a sense of trust and confidence is built up between the persons. This is the gift of defusing.[4]

8) Modeling

Modeling is emulating wealth creators. When Napoleon Hill modeled the secret of wealth accumulation and discovered what he called the Carnegie secret, he said that he found no quality *save persistence* in those who had accumulated vast fortunes. "... persistence, concentration of effort, and definiteness of purpose, were the major sources of their achievements" (p. 164).

He also noticed the power of a master mind group for reshaping one's character. Hill sought to imitate the nine men whose lives and life-works

had been most impressive to him.
> "These nine men were Emerson, Paine, Edison, Darwin, Lincoln, Burbank, Napoleon, Ford, and Carnegie. Every night, over a long period of yeas, I held an imaginary council meeting with this group whom I called my "Invisible Counselors."" (p. 215)

He spoke about studying "the records of their lives with painstaking care," and identifying with them until they became "apparently real" to him. This describes the power of having mentors (real or imagined) as well as working with and through colleagues and merging your mind with the minds of others to coordinate effort and knowledge, in a spirit of harmony. Do this to multiply your brain power. Carnegie "attributed his entire fortune to the power he accumulated through this 'Master Mind.'" (p. 170).

9) Networking
To become a collaborative wealth creator, you will want to cast your net wide so that it embraces a great many people from whom you can choose to select collaborative partners. That's what networking is about—meeting with people of like mind, discovering others with whom there might be a mutual advantage for working together, and knowing people with skills that might be useful exchange.

Obviously, you do better in any domain of effort within which you seek to achieve excellence when you have others who are like-minded and supportive. The social support that emerges when men and women of like mind, get together for networking, brainstorming, encouragement, accountability, etc. provides yet another frame that supports you.

My Personal Story
Who will go with me? Among my business partners for many years in real estate was Janine, a lady I eventually discovered when looking at a house. She was so skilled in asking questions to find my criteria and then using those to make choices, that I eventually ended up buying and selling a dozen houses through her. And once, while in Australia, she called, talked about a particular house as an investment property, and I bought it sight unseen! That was the level of trust I had in her. Then sadly she moved to Salt Lake City. Well, sad for me. Good for others!

Regarding my publishing company, *Neuro-Semantic Publications,* I worked with a printer for nearly 20 years. During those years we have a profitable win/win arrangement. Later as he become more successful, his style changed— he kept details secret, took longer and longer to respond, and would promise deliveries and dates and continually *not* make them. I can understand someone getting busy, but not continuing to make promises and not fulfill them especially after being confronted about it. Eventually I had to fire him. Like Donald Trump, one day I pointed my finger at him and said, "You're fired!"

In my work as an international trainer, I work with the association of Trainers who have come together from the shared vision of Neuro-Semantics. When it all began in 1996 I had no idea that I was, at the same time, creating an association of trusted colleagues. I had no idea that I was putting together an international association of people who would be the ones to later sponsor events for me all around the world.

In my training business I currently have, and have had, lots and lots of people who take on the role of event sponsors. At the beginning I never suspect that such would be a problem or that I would encounter incompetent sponsors. But I did. Slowly I learned how to ask questions and find people who were competent in managing and marketing an event. Then I didn't suspect that an event sponsor would possibly be unethical in handling money, but again, I learned that there were some like that and had to learn how to again ask hard questions before beginning a business relationship.

Your Adventure in Creating Wealth
So, who will go with you? Who will you share in creating wealth? Who will you make rich as you become rich? Who will make you rich as you collaborate with them? Do you need to establish your self-esteem on an unconditional basis so you don't compare yourself with others competitively? If so, review the section on "Beyond Competitiveness."

Use your *Wealth Creation Journal* to make a list of the roles and positions that need to be filled in order for your wealth creation plan to be completed. What roles, positions, skills, etc. do you need to supplement the contribution and value that you add?

Next, write out a list of your criteria for partners. I presented mine earlier which you can check out for comparison (pp. 151-152). What is your style of operating and what criteria of values and operational styles are important to you?

End of Chapter Notes:

1. See *Self-Actualization Psychology* (2008) for a full description of theory X and theory Y of management.

2. See chapter 11 on Trust in *Unleashing Leadership* (2009).

3. See *Communication Magic* (2001) which is the book about the basic NLP communication model, the Meta-Model of Language.

4. There are two chapters in *Games Great Lovers Play* (chapters 12 and 13) that translate the confrontation skills for couples, "How to Have a Really Good Fight." See the training manual on *Defusing Hotheads and other Cranky People*.

Chapter 10

CAN I MAKE A BUSINESS OUT OF THIS?

"Ownership of a business is the base upon which most people become independently wealthy." Thomas Stanley (p. 107)

"Most millionaires who take risks do many things to increase the odds of winning... they own and invest in their own businesses, they find the right niche, they do a lot of homework before investing, they love their career or business." (160-162)
Thomas Stanley (2000)

Making lots of money is one thing; creating a business that generates lots of money for you and many others, is an entirely different thing. It corresponds to Robert Kiyosaki's Cashflow Quadrants which persuasively identifies that to create wealth that will make you financially independent requires that you move from the left side of these income quadrants (from being only an employee or self-employed) to the right side where you can create and own a business and become an investor.

It is now time to talk about *creating a business* out of your wealth creation activities. Can you do that? Will you do that? If your answer to these questions is yes, then what's next? What's required to find or invent a business for your singularity? The answer to this takes us to two sets of skills that by themselves are opposites on *the Meaning—Performance Axes* which is why they do not easily and naturally go together in the same body. One set of skills enables you to become an entrepreneur; the other set enables you to become a business owner.

The set of skills for the posture, attitude, and position of being both require an unique synthesis. That's what this chapter is about: *How to be both an entrepreneur and a business owner* and how to detail the needed specifics for making it successful. So first we will explore the specialized skills of entrepreneur-ing. Then we'll look at the opposite skill, that of meta-detailing. One sets the vision, the other translates the vision to reality. Both are required for making a business out of your wealth creation passion.

> **Synergizing Entrepreneur-ing and Meta-Detailing**
>
> *1) Entrepreneur* creating a business, seeing and seizing opportunities and taking smart risks.
>
> *2) Business owner* systemizing the business, taking care of the details of the business via meta-detailing.

Side I: Entrepreneur-ing

To be an entrepreneur, you've got to have a vision—a dream. An entrepreneur is the person who sees a problem, gets excited about it, studies it, and figures out a solution for it. Essentially, an entrepreneur is a person who solves problems for a profit. So to be an entrepreneur, you have to be proactive, responsible, and have a strong belief in yourself and your passion to solve some problem (or problems). Then you have to have the commitment to take the risks of implementation that makes it happen.

Entrepreneurs are big-picture people who have eyes to *see* opportunities. The entrepreneur looks for possibilities for his or her talents and skills and when he or she sees it, is fully willing to take a risk. An entrepreneur is not emotionally dependent on money, but instead trusts in his or her mind and wits. The entrepreneur believes in creativity,

> "So the true meaning of 'entrepreneurial material' is that in spite of fear, there is the courage to 'go it alone,' to learn. Successful entrepreneurs deal with and overcome their fears."

possibilities, that loves a challenge, loves to play/work hard, and thinks long-term. Even the brightest people will never see an opportunity staring them in the face—if they're not structured for it.

Developing the Eyes of an Entrepreneur
The inside-out wealth of an entrepreneur requires that you are able to see solutions to problems and then seize market opportunities for adding that value. From there you develop the higher levels of your mind for seeing beyond and behind what's in your eyes to possibilities and opportunities. That then allows you to build the gestalt state of *seizing opportunities* that is just right for you.

If you live in a capitalistic society, then you are surrounded by lots and lots of opportunities. So to take advantage of the economic system you live in requires that you take your money and use it as capital. And that necessitates *seeing* what doesn't yet exist, but what you believe you can create.

> "Seeing opportunities that others do not see was also rated as being more important by more millionaires than 'having a high IQ/superior intellect." (Stanley, 2000, p. 62)

Seeing opportunities is a sixth sense. It is a sense that many others (probably most others) do not see. Even if you see great opportunities, it takes courage to capitalize on them because that entails selling your ideas to others. Stanley and Danko (1996) in *The Millionaire Next Door* write that entrepreneurial wealth creators "are proficient in targeting market opportunities" (p. 163).

While that's great, there's a problem. The problem is that you cannot see opportunities with your physical eyes. They are not seen in that way. *Opportunities* are not a sensory based experiences that can be literally seen, heard, or felt. You see and hear and feel "opportunities" with your mind—with your higher levels of mind. In wealth creation you need to be able to look at the events of everyday life that you might otherwise view as boring, problematic, stressful, stupid, etc., and format your thinking so that you see "opportunities" for fun, profit, development, adventure, etc.

How do you do this? You do this by meta-stating yourself with the resources of your ideas and understandings that imagines new possibilities. This creative thinking plays around with wild and crazy possibilities. Only then will a new gestalt state emerge. Begin by imagining "possibilities," "a great future," and so on.

Why do entrepreneurs do this? Yes, for the money, but always for more than just money. They have a dream and a vision that extends beyond money. Alan Anixter, president of a billion dollar wire and cable manufacturing company says that it is important to set some non-financial purposes for the business that you create.

> "Focusing on money prevents everything else from falling into place. Build a good business—the money will come along as a result."

How do you learn to "see" opportunities? First, identify a situation where you want to be able to see opportunities. When or where in creating wealth do you most need the ability to see opportunities? What situation tempts you to be blind and deaf opportunities?

Next, apply all the optimism you can access to that situation and then, as you imagine that referent and access the de-contamination of learned optimism. This will help you to *stop* seeing things through a frame of hurt or pain. When you do that, does that frame of mind now enable you to see opportunities? If so, you've got it.

If not, then the question is what mental, emotional, or personal resource do you need in order to be able to open up "the eyes of your mind?" To find out, playfully experiment with bringing some other resourceful states of mind/emotion/body to the trigger. What ideas, thoughts, beliefs, values, understandings, feelings, etc. do you need to build the mental matrix where you can "see opportunities" all around you?

After modeling many entrepreneurs, the menu list that I start with, and recommend, for the seeing opportunities include the following:

Possibility thinking	Outrageousness
Curiously wondering	Possibility thinking
Excited about problems	Pretending
Experimentation	Imagining "as if"
Problem Solving Skills	Knowledge seeker
Adventure/ Fun	Detective skills
Playfulness	Openness

To begin, take the one that you think might do the job, access that state of mind, and apply it to yourself. Second, ask yourself, the question, "How does this resource settle within me as I imagine now seeing my

situation with this mind-set? Does it create within me the eyes of an entrepreneur?"
> If so, do you like this? And if you do, and if you want to keep it, how will you do that?
>
> How will you make this a way of looking at your situation and have it available whenever you need it?

Your answer to this will give you a ritual for that resource.

The Hands of an Entrepreneur

It is not enough to *see*; you have to *seize*. It's not enough to have the eyes of an entrepreneur, *you also have to have the hands and feet of an entrepreneur.* You have to be willing to act, experiment, and implement your ideas. This is the performance axis. There are lots of visionary people walking around dreaming wonderful dreams about possibilities, but never taking the required actions to translate that vision into real-life behaviors. That's the difference that makes an effective entrepreneur.

How do you develop the ability to seize an opportunity? The first thing is, of course, having the ability to see opportunity when a problems occurs. Are you able to immediately go into an optimistic interpretative style? Take a moment to make an evaluation about how strong and available your optimism state is: How well do you see opportunities all around you? Do you need to refresh the *seeing* opportunities meta-state? If so, go back two pages and do that.

Next, you will need to identify the component elements that are the variables for the state of *seizing* opportunities. What do you need to generate the perspective and frame of mind that allows you to seize an opportunity? What criteria will you use to determine what to seize?

Again, after modeling numerous entrepreneurs for what enables them to seize opportunities, the menu list of possibilities that I use for generating *the seizing* are the following:

- Fittingness
- Time: sense of Timing
- Vision
- Values— Criteria
- Priorities
- Constraints
- Time to process
- Permission to seize

Permission to end deliberation
Decision Making:
> What am I evaluating and weighing?
> How clear are the pros and cons?

Risk management skills and style
Boldness, daring
Testing and experimenting: small test steps reality testing: prototype
Willingness to act on a possibility

As you use this list as a checklist, identify the resource you need to access them, then apply it to yourself. As you then try each resource, notice if you like it. Would this resource or resources enable you to now effectively and ecologically *seize* the opportunities that are right for you? If so, then imagine moving through life with this attitude in the weeks and months to come and notice what happens.

Side 2: Business Detailing for Watching the Store

The backside of the entrepreneurial set of skills is a special kind of detailing. It is not merely getting down to specifics, it is meta-detailing. And what is meta-detailing?

> *Meta-detailing is identifying the critical details of a activity or project from a higher or meta-perceptive.*

Meta-detailing enables you to identify *which details are important* from the perspective of the higher level principle, understanding, concept, rule, or guideline. The result enables you to delve down into details—the right details, those critical for the task, and to not get lost in irrelevant details.

By meta-detailing, you develop the ability to combine and synthesize inductive and deductive thinking, perceiving the whole *and* the specific details. You can think in global ways *and* specifically. You can *zoom in* on a picture and *zoom out*. You can *foreground* a sound or sensation and *background* others. You can *chunk up* to handle larger units of information and to get a larger perspective as well as *chunking down* to very small and even tiny bits. You can use the *precision language model* and *pull apart* a linguistic model of the world. You can also use hypnotic language to construct new enhancing realities. Putting these facets together, you facilitate a new synthesis to create *meta-detailing*.[1]

A master in a field sorts for, pays attention to, and recognizes the critical and relevant details from a meta-position. Whether a trained or a natural skill, the master recognizes and operates from some meta-pattern or principle which empowers him or her to see, hear, and sense the richness of details. This is *meta-detailing*.

With meta-detailing you are also able to balance the nobler and pettier aspects of work so you don't discount anything as "beneath" you. Without this skill it is easy to become scornful of small details. Blotnick described those in his longitudinal study:

> **The Meta-Detailing Principle:**
> The meta-frames of the big picture—of our global understandings, brilliant ideas, and key principles have to be detailed down to specific everyday activities in order to effectively implement a task or project.

"Those who found the minor details of their work a major annoyance did not persist, and became wealthy significantly less often." (p. 61)

In Blotnick's research, those who succeeded in becoming wealthy were *willing to handle both the nobler and pettier aspects.* They did the "dirty work," the trivial details and minor tasks—they didn't think anything connected with their work as "beneath" them. Blotnick:

"It will distress many to realize it, but work is 95 percent details. Far from being appalled by that fact, those who became millionaires either delighted in the details or (more often) never noticed them at all. Since the pettier aspects constitute so large a portion of each day's work, in dismissing them with a sneer you may find your life has become empty." (p. 85)

The single greatest obstacle people had in finding work that they enjoyed was their own snobbery. They would not do work "below them." The loss of status, in their minds, was too important for them (p. 241). They thought, "What will people say?" Their snooty stance is based upon a question which frightened them. Snobbery accumulates little by little and then takes away our freedom of choice.

Donald Trump (2004) speaks to this same dynamic:
"Here's something else about God that any billionaire knows: He's in

the details, and you need to be there, too." (p. xiv) "You have to be insane about the details or the whole enterprise will fail." (p. 33)

This describes the business intelligence of "watching the store." As you develop your *business smarts* about your field, laws, taxes, contracts, selling, marketing, cooperating, negotiating, building a support team—you learn how to meta-detail the specific facets of your business. Knowledge, only *potential* power, only becomes *power* when you *organize it into definite plans of action and then implement those plans.*

In meta-detailing you take a great idea and detail the specifics to create an action plan of what to do to actualize what you know. This synthesis skill is one of the hidden prerequisites of genius itself. Do so and you'll increase your creative intelligence.

About Hill, *Empire Builder of the Northwest* (1996),
"His genius lay precisely in his ability to master details while fashioning broad vision and strategy."

"Good fund managers have to be able to immerse themselves in minutiae one moment, zoom out, and look at the big picture from thirty thousand feet, then dive back into the details again." (Fortune Mag. Dec. 29, 1997, B. O'Reilly)

Meta-detailing refers to the emergent state (or gestalt) of detail processing from the perspective of a meta-concept. It involves seeing, hearing, discerning and differentiating crucial details using meta-level frames.

Meta-Detailing gives you the ability to see the big picture of your wealth creation and then to zoom down to take care of the necessary details by which you make it happen. In this way, you do not get caught up in or lost in the details. You operate from a higher sense of where you stand with things, what you are doing, why you are doing them, what you seek to achieve. This keeps your work with details clean. Otherwise you might forget where you are and what you're doing. Otherwise you might go off on tangents and side-alleys and get lost. Otherwise, you would not be able to discern a *trivial* detail from a *critical* one.

In this way, meta-detailing enables you to stay focused, directed, insightful, and persistent. It enriches your abilities to make decisions.

Having a higher sense of how various details play into the larger picture enables you to operate from an almost intuitive "knowing" about what is truly important and what is not.

Meta-detailing saves you from living in the clouds with great plans and tremendous visions, but lacking the practical knowledge of how to take care of the details. Visionaries often suffer because they develop "a bad relationship" to details. The person who says, "I'm a global person; I don't do details" will also be a person who probably will *not* develop expertise and excellence in their field.

Meta-Detailing Supports Patience and Persistence
In the domain of wealth creation, Blotnick (1980) noticed how a poor relationship to details undermines a person's ability to succeed. Such an attitude typically arises from some other attitudes and states (impatience, greediness, dislike of work, etc.) that further undermine success.

> "His intense desire to be a wealthy executive made him scornful of small details of any sort. 'Why should I have to deal with this sort of crap?' he asked exasperatedly. Unfortunately, petty details are an essential and abundant part of every aspect of business.
>
> "Their existence therefore isn't the real issue. Your response to them is. You can make a mountain out of any molehill, if you want to. And what we discovered is that someone is likely to do precisely that if they don't happen to like their job. In fact, the more they disliked it, the more resentful they are likely to be about its petty details. To put it more positively: people who enjoy their work usually didn't notice the many details connected with each task they had to attend to." (p. 60)

By way of contrast, he spoke about some of *the meta-frames* of values, beliefs, understandings, ideas, decisions, etc. that would enable and enrich the details.

> "It gave Rita enormous satisfaction to do her job well. In a business in which even minor errors may look major to customers, Rita enjoyed seeing quality work produced. 'We don't always do it flawlessly,' she said, but she was indeed prepared to try." (Blotnick, p. 61)

The problem with people who find the minor details of their work a major annoyance is that they simply do not persist. And without persistence, they became wealthy significantly less often.

> "Neither focusing solely on the details nor ignoring them altogether is wise. Something in between is obviously called for. And strangely enough, the people who accidently located that Golden Mean were

those who profoundly enjoyed doing their work. Their absorption in it also allowed time to pass far more quickly than it did for others." (p. 68)

The details you will want to notice and handle in creating wealth include specifics about finances, book keeping, quality control over product and services, dealing effectively with customer satisfaction, employees, investments, real estate, taxes, etc. Are you ready to go there? Do you have sufficient meta-frames to do so?

Detailing Business Success
First, identify three to five principles that govern success, excellence, expertise, or mastery in your business. Are you ready to do this from business? Great. What do the experts in your field know that creates their competitive edge or expertise? What principles, concepts, understandings enrich and enhance their performances? What frames of mind are involved in these or are presupposed in these? What higher frames make up the rules in their game?

Second, fully express one of these principles. Write it out in full until you have a clear expression of it. Be precise to state it with such crystal clarity that it immediately makes sense to someone unfamiliar with your field. Rewrite it until you can describe the principle with both clarity and succinctness. Rewrite again until the clear and succinct statement feels compelling to you.

Third, step into the state that the principle evokes. As you read and feel the principle that you've clarified, made succinct and compelling, see, hear and feel it. Experience it fully in the context of your work. Identify one specific behavior that corresponds to this principle—that enables you to express the principle through that behavior. The behavior would fit and be congruent with the principle. Repeat until you see-hear-feel 5 to 10 details that give flesh-and-blood to the principle.

Imagine stepping into the details to experience doing them. As you do so, go meta to the principle that governs these details. From within your vivid imagery of the detailing, shift upward to the governing principle that drives and organizes the details. Now open your eyes and ears to experience your world from the meta-level of the detailing. Repeat this several times to create a synergy of the meta-principle and the detail that actualizing it.

Finally, enrich with resources and future pace. What resources do you need to make these details more important, memorable, and compelling? What resources would enrich you so that you are the kind of person who takes care of these details?

The Business of Business
In addition to business detailing (what I've been calling *meta-detailing*), there are several other key business skills for creating wealth. These include selling yourself and your products and services, taking risks in a smart way, and handling taxes.

> **The Selling Principle:**
> Wealth is created by selling ourselves, our ideas, our products, and our services.

The Business Skill of Selling
What's involved in business, in creating a business, running a business, and maintaining an efficient business? A deceiving myth is that if you have something of great value, the world will somehow hear about it, will somehow spontaneously know who you are and where you are, and with that beat a path to your door. And while that would be great, it doesn't work that way. *You have to sell.*

You have to find or create a market for what you offer of value. Not only is this a prerequisite for creating wealth, you are already involved in selling anyway. After all, as an employee, you sell yourself to an employer to hire you, to give you raises and promotions, and to believe in your value. The question is not whether you sell, the question is: *What is your skill level when you sell?* Do you mindfully focus on improving yourself in this area? As an employee, you have a customer. We all do. You have customers that need to be persuaded, sold, influenced, and treated with top-notch customer service. You have to get the word out.[2]

A Selling Exploration:
1) Object:
       What do you sell?
       And what else?
2) Target:
       To whom do you sell?
       Who are all of your customers and clients?
       What market are you selling within?

What other markets could you expand to?
What are you products and services?
What are the key features that you have to offer?
What are the benefits and meta-benefits of those features?

3) Theme and benefits:
What is your unique selling point (proposition)?
Why should they buy from you?
What do you have to offer? And what else?

4) Skill:
How skillful are you in marketing, selling, and influencing?
How much fun do you have in doing so?
How much more fun, charming, playful, and resourceful could you make it?
Are you willing to improve your skills and attitude in this area?
What do you need in order to do that?

The Business of Risk Taking

Are you ready and able to capitalize your business? How does the world of finances, saving, budgeting, investing, business, creating wealth, marketing, creating alliances, etc. work? To navigate this territory, you will need to develop a well-formed understanding about all of the facets of money.

Capitalizing on your finances through budgeting, saving, frugality, planning, increasing sources of income, etc. enables you to build capital. You can *not* create wealth if you are spending impulsively, up to your neck in debt, and unable to master your finances. Financial self-control is an essential step in order to build a system where money can work for you instead of you working for money.

If you are confident about your dream and your skills, then you focus everything into a singular concentrate in this stage of building your business. This is not the time to diversify. Robert Allen says that in the first stage of wealth building is the time to concentrate all of your eggs in the right basket.

Robert Kiyosaki (1996) frames diversification as an investment strategy for "not losing." It is not an investment strategy for winning. In his experience, successful investors do not diversify, they focus their efforts.

"We believe that a policy of portfolio concentration may well decrease risk if it raises both the intensity with which an investor thinks about a business and the comfort level he must feel with its economic characteristics before buying into it." (p. 43)

The Business Skill of Handling Taxes

Taxes and penalties can eat up both your income and your capital. To avoid this you will want to develop your financial intelligence about taxes and tax opportunities. The overall strategy will be to minimize your taxable income and maximize your unrealized income (wealth or capital appreciation without a cash flow). So if that's your strategy, how will you use your financial intelligence to understand how to take advantage of any and every tax benefit. How will you attain that knowledge? Who will you work with?

> **The Tax Principle**
>
> Wealth is created by reducing our taxes in every way that's possible and legal (especially legal)! Wealth is created by paying for good legal and tax advice. Get a good accountant.

If you are to keep your expectations well-adjusted to tax reality, as Robert Allen suggests, then do not count your dollars until you have passed them through the strainer of taxes and inflation. Then as you recognize the role of both taxes and inflation in your wealth creation plans, you will be more able to take effective actions to reduce taxes legally and to use instruments and processes that will help.

Investing Your Wealth

After you have money to invest, how do you invest your money intelligently so that money works for you instead of you for money?

Just as the get-rich-quick mentality undermines, interferes, and sabotages with the creation of wealth and financial independence, so it also undermines intelligent and productive investments.

In Blotnick's language, the Stage Two orientation, namely, to first get rich, then decide on your passions and lifestyle, can cause you to desperately want to become rich so much that you engage in impulsive and unwise investing. And when that happens, you end up making poor decisions about your investments and possibly losing all of your hard-earned money.

"Investments" and Mad Meanings

What is an "investment" anyway? If you equate "investment" with "good value for money" the very confusion of that definition will undermine your investment success. "Good value for money" is not a definition of investment! At best, it is a definition of intelligent purchasing.

If you equate "investment: with consumption, you create madness. Why? Because you will then begin to try to "spend your way to riches." Think about that! If you equate investment with spending, it is an easy and slippery slope to begin thinking that you can spend your way to riches!

Yet the reasoning become circular:
>Why do you want to become rich?
>>"To spend it, of course!"
>And how are you going to become rich?
>>"By investing."

What all of this creates a state of impulsive investing. Like crazed hunters who shoot at anything that moves, so crazed investors throw their money away at anything called an "investment." But fun investments, and consumption investments are not truly investments. "Saving" creates tremendous confusion. Yet the advertizement is everywhere: "Save 50 percent off the sticker price today!" Of course, spending to (so-call) "invest" can blind you to the fact that you are actually spending.

The Art of Investing Wisely?
How do you go about investing wisely? There are several steps.

1) Decide on your risk quotient.
How much can you risk to lose? How bold or cautious do you want to be when you are investing your money? Set a limit so that you know what you can and cannot afford. Then take time to thoughtfully encounter what it would be like to lose that investment. If you are still okay with life and yourself if that happened, then you at least have faced the "worst case scenario."

2) Learn the critical success factors of investment.
What are the critical factors that make for success in investing? First and

foremost, know the product or company in which you are investing. Do your homework to study the market and the product. Study the company— how is it led, how managed, how are the people recruited, trained, coached, and treated?

3) Identify your trust level.
How much do you trust the information that you have received? How much do you trust the product, the company, and the leadership? How much do you trust yourself in this process?

My Personal Story
The first business I consciously created for creating wealth was my real estate investments. At the time, I believed that I could make much more money in real estate rather than in training. So that's where I put my focus. While researching and training was my love, I applied my learnings to understand real estate as the business and how to effectively work with people. I did all of that in service of creating the financial independence I wanted.

After getting involved in that business, I found a new passion— finding and working with the renters. My objective and goal was to find good responsible people who wanted to live in one of my houses and who also wanted to take care of it. I wanted people who would responsibly take care of the property and people who recognized the value I was providing in a clean, affordable home, with the possibility of home ownership.

This led to my real estate business—to buying and selling houses. I began at the lower end of the housing market and within a few short years moved to the middle of that market. For many years, the investment grew at the rate of 10 to 18 percent per year. By the late 1990s I was only buying brand new houses (three and four bedroom homes) and doing so on 15 year loans. The business model that I used was to put 15 to 20 percent down. Then the family renting the house would pay for the mortgage. In the United states, the interest paid on the mortgage went to reduce my taxes. And every improvement in the property achieved two goals—it pleased those renting and it increased the value of the property.

As all of this was happening, my work in the field of training and development was also growing. As my skills increased, so did my reputation for excellence in getting results with groups. Within a few years, I was making more money than I ever dreamed possible. And that, in turn, gave me more time to focus on my international training business. Eventually, I had to increase my fees just to manage the demand on my time. Then as I developed processes for others to do the same trainings, I created a simple and modest way to receive royalties from the training manuals. This turned my previous work into a source of passive income and contributed to my financial independence.

Your Adventure in Creating Wealth
As your Wealth Coach, I now get to do some business coaching with you. Are you ready?

Question 1: Can you create a business out of your passion and competencies? If so, what business? Do you have a business plan for it? How well developed is that plan? Have you written out your Matrix Business Plan for it?[3] Will you do that this week?

Question 2: What is your business model? What is the value that you add to your customers or clients? How will you communicate that value to them? How will you brand that value? Who is your market? What are their characteristics and demographics? What is the profit margin between expenses and income?

Question 3: Who are your competitors? What will differentiate you from them? What are the best practices of your competitors? What can you learn from their best practices?

Question 4: Are you an entrepreneur? Are you willing to develop your skills in entrepreneuring? Do you need to focus mostly on seeing or seizing opportunities?

Question 5: How are you at meta-detailing the specifics of your business? If you need to change or expand your global meta-program, see *Figuring Out People,* chapter 11.

End of Chapter Notes

1. I first discovered meta-detailing when I was working on the book, *Sub-Modalities Going Meta* (1999/2003). That's when I discovered that meta-detailing is a key element in the structure of genius.

2. See the training manual, "Selling Genius."

3. We use the Matrix Business Plan in Meta-Coaching and other trainings. Simply use the eight distinctions of the Matrix Model and ask a dozen questions about it using your *business* as the subject.

PART III

THE STATES OF

WEALTH CREATION

To create wealth you have to access and operate from the right state. And there are numerous right states. Some are primary states, some are meta-states, and some are the emergent gestalt states.

Chapter 11

WHAT ARE THE BEST STATES FOR WEALTH CREATION?

> "If you learn how to manage your states and your behaviors, you can change anything."
> Anthony Robbins (1986, p. 321)

> *"Your emotional state ultimately determines your financial state."*
> Suze Orman (p. 11)

Wealth creation is all about state. Your ability to create wealth and to do so year after year ultimately requires that you access and operate from your best states. *State* grounds your meanings, beliefs, and indeed—your whole Matrix of frames. No wonder we have covered a great many states in the previous chapters. It is now time to specifically focus on state as one of the secrets of inside-out wealth. *Rich robust states* offer you a process, a means and a context, for creating wealth.

How are you at accessing the following states? Gauge from 0 to 10 how skilled and able you are to access and operate from the following states at will and to use them to support your wealth creation:
__ Intention and Purpose
__ Focus
__ Decision
__ Commitment
__ Passion
__ Self-Mastery
__ Patience
__ Persistence
__ Valuing

__ Empowerment
__ Execution; implementation
__ Self-Acceptance
__ Self-Confidence
__ Self-Esteem
__ Self-Efficacy
__ Learning; Curiosity
__ Creativity
__ Joy; fun
__ Frugality
__ Integrity
__ Collaboration
__ Risk taking
__ Detailing
__ Seeing Opportunities
__ Seizing Opportunities

> **The State Principle:**
> Wealth is created by operating from the right states. If you can't manage your mind and states, what makes you think you can manage your money? To succeed in business and in wealth creation, identify your best states for you for creating wealth and then operate out of the right states.

The Composition of States

A state is made up of various mental and physical ingredients. A powerful mind-body-emotion (or neuro-linguistic) state contains powerful supporting ideas, beliefs, values, representations along with empowering physiology that keeps you focused and energized. And as mind-body experiences, states are holistic, circular, cybernetic, determinative, and habitual.

Linguistically (that is, in language) we can separate mind, body, and emotion, yet this gives the false impression that they are separate entities. They are not. Your mind-body system, as mine, works as a whole. That's what *state* is. This also explains why the term *state* is more holistic and useful then to speak about "mind," "body," or "emotion" implying that they are separate things. They are not.

The mind component of a state refers to your thinking, representing, imagination, memory, framing, etc. What ideas can you entertain that will put you into that state? How do you internally represent an idea so that it evokes that state? After you identify a state for creating wealth that you want to access and operate from, identify the ideas and their corresponding physiology needed to access that state. *The body component* of a state refers to your physiology, kinesthetics, and neurology. What physical movements, gestures, postures, etc. correspond to that state?

The emotion component of a state refers to how your mind and body sensations ("feelings" and kinesthetics) combine to create your "emotions." An emotion is a somatic response to your meanings which activates your physiology. An emotion literally activates you so that you "move out" and generates an "action tendency" of response.[1]

As you undoubtedly have already realized, for wealth creation, you will need different states for different activities.
- What are your top wealth creation states?
- What states do you need to earn, save, and invest money wisely?
- What states do you need in order to work with and through others?
- What states do you need to do your best when you are at work?
- What states do you need to manage your money effectively (budget, save, invest, etc.)?

Your Wealth Profile
Have you identified your best wealth creation states? If so, you have taken the first step. Having done that, do you also know how to access them effectively? You can use the list of states at the beginning of this chapter as a checklist of great states to access as you create wealth. What are the states of mind that you will need to attract riches?

It's one thing to know that your states can help you create and attract wealth, it's another thing to have the skill of accessing, building, and maintaining such states. As you make a list of your top ten states for discovering and creating the kind of wealth that you want, consider the attitude and character these states create within you because it is the combination and synergy of your states that create your style. One of the most critical states for the right attitude that you will need is *the state of abundance* about life, yourself, etc. Operate from abundance and you will be able to take the right actions that will create wealth.

Accessing and Managing your Best States
The biggest challenge that faces all of us, whether in wealth creation or in life, is managing our moods and attitudes—that is our *states*. Your rich, robust wealth creation states are your foundation for creating inside-out wealth. *Your best states are your best assets.* Do you know that? Are you ready to mind-to-muscle that principle?
"I will make my states dynamic, dramatic, powerful, playful, etc.

When I do that, then it will be easy to sell myself on it!"

Top Wealth Creation States
— Caring, loving, passionate
— Passionately committed: engaged, absorbed
— A sense of personal mission
— Invincible, tenacious
— Initiation, proactive,
— Patient, long-term perspective
— Response-able
— Cooperative, collaborative, empathetic
— Self-investment — Self-disciplined
— Flexible, adaptable — Adventurous
— Reality oriented
— Playful: sense of humor, cheerful
— Tolerant of discomfort and anxiety
— Courage (to invest, take risks)
— Respect and honor
— Perceptual flexibility
— Authenticity: being real, Integrity
— Open: willingness to experiment
— Strong, energetic
— Appreciative, thankful
— Excited/ enthusiastic — Generous
— Vital, vigorous — Empowered
— Flirtatious: warm, friendly, outgoing

What Meta-States did you choose for Wealth Building?
__ Curious attention to detail
__ Attentive listening for new ideas
__ Playful earnestness
__ Joyful commitment
__ Meta-detailing
__ Willingness to take wise and informed risks
__ Tolerance of discomfort
__ Centered in clear visions and values
__ Courage
__ Refusing to play it safe
__ Intelligently risking
__ Refusing to be pushed around by financial conditions
— Balanced
— Self-control: Executive choice
— Self-integrity: living by higher values and motives

> **States that are Ineffective:**
> — Impatience
> — Greed
> — Fear
> — Fearful, worrisome
> — Timidity
> — Insecurity
> — Revenge
> — Overly Ambitious
> — Competitive
> — Peevish
> — Consumption-oriented
> — Boredom
> — Easily frustrated
> — Negativity, pessimism
> — Procrastination
> — Regret
> — Perfectionism
> — Overwhelmed
> — Arrogant
> — Critical, judgmental
> — Stressed out
> — Snobbish

The Art of Accessing Your Best States

What is the process for identifying, developing, accessing, and solidifying your best states for wealth creation? Begin by identifying your best desired state and its mind-body components. What state do you want? If you find someone to describe that state to, you will discover the amazing power that you have in just verbally describing the state. Notice what that does for you. The amazing thing is that by describing the state, you call it forth. Describing it enables you also to enter into it. As you focus on how you represent that state, do you now recognize one mechanism you can use to access it at will? I hope so.

Evoking a state can occur through three different avenues. First, you can use *memory* to access a state. The formula in NLP is: "Think of a time when you fully experienced this state..." That is, recall a time when you clearly had it in a powerful way. What thoughts really evoke this state for you? What do you need to do to really crank up this state? How much do you now have the feeling of this state? As the feelings emerge, take a moment to simply be with those feelings ... let them grow ... now double the intensity of those feelings ... What would increase the experience of this state even more?

A second way to access a state is to *use your imagination.* The formula is this: "What would it be like if you were fully experiencing this state?" And if that doesn't do it for you, then *use the modeling question:* "Do you know anyone who has ever experienced that state? How did they look, act, what did that person say? Now imagine becoming that person for a moment; what is that like?

After you have accessed the state, the way to keep it so you have ready access to it at any time is to "anchor" it. Anchor your state when you have amplified the state so that you are experiencing it fully in your body. Then link some stimuli to it—an image, sound, touch, movement. You can use a physical touch on the arm, forearm, or shoulder when you reach the peak of the state. Or you can anchor it visually through a gesture or auditorially by a particular tone of voice.

Let's say you have the state, have anchored it, now practice stepping in and out of that state. That is, break your state and then re-access it again. As you do this several times, it gives you a sense of control and ownership of the state.[2]

Next, apply this resourceful state to a time or place when you need it in your everyday life. Where could you really use this state on a daily basis as you engage in various wealth creation activities? Think of that time and *feel this* (fire the anchor — trigger the stimulus you've connected to the state). Suppose you had this feeling or way of thinking as your attitude, fully and completely, in just the way that you would want it —would you like that? Would that attitude transform things as you think about that activity? How would it transform things ... just notice inside ... and enjoy. [A suggestion: Have someone take you through this process so that you can fully experience it.]

Powerful Wealth Creation Gestalt States
The *meta-stating process* refers to working methodically with your consciousness—with your self-reflexive consciousness—to utilize the

spiraling and looping of your mind as you react to your reactions. This enables you to feed back into your consciousness new awarenesses to give you more choice, grace, elegance, and resourcefulness. When you do this time and again within your neuro-semantic system, a new emergent properties arise. These higher emergent states are what we call *gestalt states.* And now that you know how to do it, you also have another avenue for creating fabulous states.

How? Knowing how to meta-state yourself now allows you to embed many meta-levels of states (or contexts) as you design new emergent frames of mind that will work optimally for you. By understanding the layering of meta-states, and the emergence of gestalt states, you now also know how to read and understand the literature in the field of wealth creation. Here are some examples.

As you read these sentences from some of the key thinkers in wealth creation, notice the "recipe" or "formula" within them. The authors wrote these originally from their own experience without knowing the Meta-States Model. But now that you know *the layering process and how to relate one resource to another to create complex states,* you can read the self-reflexive structure implied in these statements. So now, instead of just hearing lots of words and great ideas, you'll be able to detect the structure that each writer recommends.

Kiyosaki offers this on wealth creating:
> "If it doesn't take money to make money, and schools do not teach you how to become financially free, then what does it take? It takes a dream, a lot of determination, a willingness to learn quickly, and the ability to use your God-given assets properly and to know which section of the Cashflow Quadrant to generate your income from."

Essentially his formula in this statement is to add a dream plus (+) determination + willingness to learn quickly + the use of your personal assets. Combine all of these together and you'll have the ideal state and strategy that he is suggesting.

Martha Sinetar writes:
> "Money is more likely to follow the person with determination, talent, and the high self-esteem that allows him to be a healthy chooser, so that his risk-taking, judgment skills, and sense of timing are sound. Money is also more likely to follow the person who has tapped into the vitality

hidden in the things he loves." (*Do What You Love and the Money will Follow,* p. 137)

Her formula in that paragraph: Determination + talent + high self-esteem + risk taking + judgment + sense of timing X (times) the vitality of something loved. That is, multiply all of these factors by the vitality of your love.

Napoleon Hill offers this highly poetic one:

> **Three kinds of States**
> 1) Primary states
> 2) Meta-states
> 3) Gestalt states

"Faith is the head chemist of the mind. When faith is blended with thought, the subconscious mind instantly picks up the vibration, translates it into its spiritual equivalent." (p. 49) Keep repeating your faith until it becomes your habit of mind.

"Every man is what he is because of the dominating thoughts which he permits to occupy his mind. Thoughts which a man deliberately places in his own mind and encourages with sympathy, and with which he mixes any one or more of the emotions, constitute the motivating forces which direct and control his every moment, act, and deed!" (p. 53)

The formula: Faith as vibration + unconscious mind translation + repetition + sympathetic encouragement + emotion.

Walt Disney writes about his success in these words:

"[Our success] was built by hard work and enthusiasm, integrity of purpose, a devotion to our medium, confidence in its future, and, above all, by a steady day-by-day growth in which we all simply studied our trade and learned."(1941, *Growing Pains*)

That gives us the following formula: Hard work + enthusiasm + integrity of purpose + devotion to medium + confidence in future X day-by-day growth.

"Our studio had become more like a school than a business. We were growing as craftsmen, through study, self-criticism, and experiment. ... Each year we could handle a wider range of story material, attempt things we would not have dreamed of tackling the year before. I claim that this is not genius or even remarkable. It is the way men build a sound business of any kind— sweat, intelligence, and love of the job." (*The Art of Walt Disney,* by C. Finch. 1973, p. 171).

Another formula: Growing craftsmen + study + self-criticism + experimentation in context of sweat + intelligence + love of the job.

Gestalting States

When you meta-state a primary state with numerous resources, you layer the first state with level upon level of other thoughts and feelings. This enables you to initiate a new gestalt and so create richer and more complex states for building wealth.

The term "gestalt" refers to a configuration of mind-and-emotion that comes together and emerges from many interactive parts in a system so that "the whole is greater than the sum of the parts." In a gestalt state you will have one or more levels of meta-states outframing a primary state. This gives rise to a new and richer experience.

Negative Emotions
— Fear
— Greed
— Perfectionism
— Negativity
— Anger
— Peevish
— Revenge
— Boredom
— Low self-value

Negative Experiences
—Competitiveness
— Shame
— Entitlement
— Snobbery
— Self-indulgence
— Laziness
— Reactive

For gestalting (or creating a complex meta-state), first identify the elements and components of this new state. Actually, this is the most challenging part of the process and may take a good bit of experimenting until you find the right component pieces that will work for you. What do you need to make up a rich and vibrant state of this experience (resilience, persistence, self-esteem, etc.)? What are the elements of optimism? The components of seeing opportunities? Of courage? How do you need to customize the state so that it creates the precise mind-set for you that feels compelling for you? What do you need to think, feel, know, value, believe so that this gestalt experience emerges for you?

Once you have all or some of the pieces, meta-state each state to the context of your primary state. That is, access the resource, amplify it to the optimal degree, and then apply to yourself. And as always with meta-states, it's best to use small and simple examples for accessing the new resource. If you are doing it by yourself, ask yourself, "What is a good reference for the first element?" Then do that with the second, the third, and so on. With each resource, check how much do you feel it; explore if you need to do to strengthen it or reduce it.

The tricky part comes when you apply that resource to your primary state or experience. The trick will be holding your referent steady so that the second thought *applies* and is *linked to* the first. After each application, check to see what happens as you apply that particular resource to the primary experience. Has the new gestalted meta-state emerged? If not, keep adding resources until it does.

When you have the state, you're now ready to appropriate it into your world. The questions I typically use to facilitate this are:
> "How would you like to *feel this* [fire the entire meta-state as a anchored resource] as you move out into your everyday life of work, career, with friends, etc.? How does that fit? Are you fully aligned with this? Any other resource do you need or want? Is it fully ecological?"

If all of your answers are yes, then you're ready to make an empowering decision to set this new meta-state. Say a meta-yes to it. Do that by saying a strong *yes* to the following questions:
> "Would you like to have this? Would this make life better? Are you willing to make this your program? How will it affect your self-definition? But how will you remember it?"[3]

Eliminating Sabotaging States

If *the right states* are crucial for creating wealth, *the wrong states* can undermine and sabotage your wealth creating abilities. As you well know, some states will powerfully work against you and your best interests in creating and accumulating wealth. If you live in these states, they will toxify your mind-and-emotions. They will contaminate and poison your power to create wealth in a healthy and ecological way. They will become "dragons" or "gremlins" to your personal success. The person who happens to make a lot of money from these states will still be a loser in the game and will suffer the emotional pain of being neurotic, unhappy, bitter, paranoid, etc.

- Are you committed to getting everything *out of the way* that's in the way of your success?
- Are you ready to deal with your conflicts, inhibitions, fears, toxic ideas, wrong states and intentions, misunderstandings, cognitive distortions, etc.?
- Are you ready to clear the path by dealing with any and all fears?
- Are you ready to learn how to refuse to give in to anything that would stop you?

Fear as a Saboteur

The primary sabotaging emotion is fear and specifically irrational fears. By its nature, fear assumes danger and threat and so will induce you into a constricting, debilitating, and nerve-wracking state. All this energy is great if there is a true danger to your physical well-being. It will not do you well if the fear is psychological. And the biggest fears among us humans are fears of rejection, failure, risk taking, and losing. These are the fears that will prevent you seeing opportunities and keep you trapped as a slave to security.

Writing about fear, Robert Kiyosaki says:
"The main reason so many people struggle financially is not because they lack a good education, or are not hard working. It's because they're *afraid* of losing. If the fear of losing stops them, they've already lost." (2000, p. 152)

Greed as a Saboteur

Always wanting more and never feeling satisfied, forever dissatisfied, so you never can say, "Enough." If you don't know when to stop, then it will be hard to say *No,* to take off, to enjoy. You'll be constantly distracted with new projects.

"Impatiently ambitious people unwittingly sell themselves on the pitch that if they act the wealthy part, that will help them to get there. It will not." (Blotnick, p. 59).

Blind or exaggerated ambition will cause you to try too hard to become rich. It will make you too needy for money and ironically, this will sabotage your wealth creation. This is also true for being highly competitive as already noted:

"The more intensely competitive someone was, the *less* likely they were to become wealthy." (Blotnick, p. 150)

"The reason that so few people are financially independent today is that *they place many negative roadblocks in their heads.* Becoming wealthy is, in fact, a mind game. And millionaires often talk to themselves about the benefits of becoming financially independent. They constantly tell themselves that it is very difficult to achieve that without taking some risks. Before you can become a millionaire, you must learn to think like one. You must learn how to motivate yourself constantly to counter fear with courage." (Stanley, 2000, p. 135)

Impatience as a Saboteur
Wanting to get rich quickly also feeds the state of impatience and will lead you to be peevish and easily annoyed. The person who overly and exclusively focuses on the grandeur will tend to have disdain for the petty details required for success. The attitude is, "If only I were rich, I wouldn't have to put up with this."

Impatience also arises from low frustration tolerance. The inability to handle stress and challenges leads to the lack of persistence. Entitlement feelings that assume that the world or your parents owe you will do the same.

> "I cringe whenever I hear people ask me how to get rich quicker." (Robert Kiyosaki)

Wrong Motives as a Saboteur
If the motive for creating wealth is toxic like trying to "be a somebody," that very motive will undermine and work as a saboteur to your success. This includes name-dropping, socializing, needing to impress people, caring too much about your impressions and reputation, etc. Self-value is *the cause* of wealth creation, not the result. Self-value creates inside-out wealth (noted in chapter 8, *Am I a Wealth Creator?*) so that you first become wealthy on the inside, then you crate wealth on the outside.

Negativity as a Saboteur
The state of thinking and seeing the world through negative lens leads to a critical and "won't work" attitude. The negativity contaminates your focus so all you can see are the downside of problems and head-aches that business brings. Living in negativity then leads to disbelieving and developing a cynicism that simply will not support you in creating wealth.

Escaping an Old Sabotaging Matrix
If your matrix of frames prevents you from creating wealth, you first need to escape that semantic field. So, how do you do that?

First, identify your wealth creation problems and situations. Then within those contexts, explore to find the specific saboteur or saboteurs.

> What stops you from creating wealth? How do you know this? What gets in your way? How does it get in your way? To what extent? What do you need in order to create wealth?

Once you know *what* the saboteur is, you are ready to explore your frames about the problem, situation, or interference. And to do that, simply go through the meaning and meta-questions:

> What do you believe about that problem or situation? What does it mean to you? How do you describe it? If that's so, then what do you believe about that? If that's true, so what?

Simply keep asking meta-questions to explore this matrix of frames. Once you have fully mapped out your old matrix of frames about the saboteur, then step back and run a quality control on the old matrix. As you step back, you can now ask these leverage questions:

> What do you think about this set of frames about creating wealth? Do these frames enhance and enrich you? Do they empower you to create wealth? Have you had enough of them? Are you ready to escape that old matrix?

If you are ready to escape the old matrix, then you are in a position to begin to imagine a whole new set of frames. So, if you could escape the old matrix and create a whole new set of frames, what would you like to think, feel, believe, understand, etc. that would enhance and empower you?

> What would you need to believe or know or understand that would support this? And what else? Continue to do this until you have a set of frames that are well-described.

The final step is to map out a set of new actions that will arise from this new way of thinking. This will comprise your action plan. If you believed all of that and you commissioned it to guide your actions, what would you be doing? What else?

My Personal Story
What are my best states for wealth creation? My best states are those of a persistent focus, creativity and the playing with ideas, a commitment to continuous improvement, learning and undefeatable curiosity, and efficiency with time and energy. These are the states that create and innovate new models and patterns in Neuro-Semantics. These are the key states that I use in trainings, business consulting, and coaching.

While preparing this text in January 2010, I was co-training in Hong Kong with Colin Cox when someone asked a very personal question. "What is your secret for being so productive?" After I attempted a feeble answer, Colin commented. He said that I was extremely disciplined and that it is the discipline that enables me to be efficiently focused in writing and other things. While that was not the answer I gave, it made perfect sense. Later I reflected about this and realized that I had always just assumed discipline as one of the requirements for getting anything done. And I suppose it is one of my best states.

For buying real estate my best states involve another set: gaining rapport, curious questioning, and negotiating. These correspond to my basic beliefs about buying and selling properties. First, it is all about relationships, so gaining *rapport* and connecting to people is essential. It's how I come to understand the people I'm doing business with. *Ferocious curiosity* because I believe that I need to understand and the only way I can really do that is by asking and by asking the most obvious and "dumb" questions. Only then can I operate from facts rather than guesses and mind-reading. And *negotiating* because I believe that everything is negotiable. Prices are set by people, they do not fall out of the heavens written on tablets of stone. Someone, somewhere, sets the price and they do it because they make an evaluation about the value of something. And if a human set the price, a human can adjust it.

Your Adventure in Creating Wealth
As your Wealth Coach, your task after this chapter is to go back over the list of states in the list earlier in this chapter and put a plus sign (+) by the following states if you feel that you already have in sufficient intensity and power. Put a minus sign (-) by those that you need to more fully develop so you have ready access to them. Which state will you work on this week? How will you cultivate that state and develop it?

What is your evidence that the state you chose is truly an effective wealth creation state? Who can you check in with to determine how well it actually serves you? How ecological are the states you have chosen?

Write your top states for creating wealth into your *Inside-Out Wealth Creation Plan.* How will you practice accessing those best states so that you have them at ready access? What is your plan for developing and practicing the states that you need to become much more effective as a wealth creator?

End of Chapter Notes

1. Originally "emotion" was spelt *ex-motion* and so indicated the *motion* that is generated that *moves* you *out (ex-)* from where you are and so creates motivational energy.

2. For a full description of the anchoring process, see *User's Manual of the Brain, Volume I.*

3. For the meta-stating process, see *Meta-States* (2008). *Secrets of Personal Mastery* (1999). Even more useful would be to attend the APG Meta-States workshop—Accessing Personal Genius.

Chapter 12

WHAT ARE THE HIGHEST STATES FOR WEALTH CREATION?

*"Those who want to become wealthy
have to learn to manage their fears and especially their fear of risk.
We have to move beyond playing it safe to playing it smart."*
Robert Kiyosaki

*"The single most important quality you need
in order to change the course of your life is courage.
A great deal of courage."*
*"It takes courage to make the decisions today
that may make us rich tomorrow."*
Suze Orman

There are states and then there are high level states— *meta-states*. These higher states arise from your self-reflexive consciousness as you reflect back onto yourself—your primary states and your experiences. This creates your layered consciousness—a mind that holds many thoughts and awarenesses at the same time in reference to the same event or experience. In this chapter we'll explore four fabulous wealth creation meta-states:
- Courage
- Persistence
- Efficiency
- Resilience

Courage as a Wealth Creation State

Courage bridges the interface between your visions and plans to the outside world thereby making real your ability to add value and make a difference. Knowing a field and developing a business is not enough. Bold and courageous actions are required to act on your knowledge and close your knowing-doing gap. This takes courage. It requires the inside-out wealth of being action-oriented, managing risk, and staying focused.

Courage (guts, chutzpah, balls, audacity, daring) is the mental or moral strength that enables you to resist opposition, danger, and hardship. Courage gives you the power and willingness to take risks, to live easily with insecurity, and to make mistakes. As a frame of mind of firmness, courage is mental or moral strength to venture, persevere, without danger, fear, or difficulty. Courage takes positive moral actions.

There are a great many acts of courage needed in the wealth creation process. Suze Orman mentions many of these in *Acts of Courage*. Her lists includes:
> To have more and to be more; to look within; to make room for more money; to value money; to face the unknown; to refuse failure; to open your heart and hands; to be rich; to create your financial destiny; to keep bouncing back.

Perhaps one of the first, and one of the scariest, acts requiring courage is the act of becoming self-employed.
> "[The self-made millionaires] are of the mind-set that it is risky *not* to be self-employed. Being self-employed means that you are in control of your own destiny. Profits that are made are yours." (Stanley, p. 18)

To take the leap, you need to be grounded in yourself, grounded in your knowledge, your skills, and the value that you add. Earlier I described this as self-efficacy— you trust yourself to be able to cope and even master a challenge. It is this state that reduces the sense of risk. After all, you are only risking time, money, and effort, not the real wealth of life.
> "Time and time again, the millionaires bolster their courage with thoughts like these: *What if I lost everything, every dollar? I would still have what's most important, my husband/wife and my children. They would never abandon me.*" (Stanley, p. 173)

As self-made millionaires are able to see opportunities that others ignore, they are willing to take financial risk after thoughtful reflection. They also willingly sell their ideas—all of this takes courage.

"Why do those who are likely to become part of the next generation of millionaires take risks today? In their minds, economic risk taking is a requirement for becoming financially independent." (200, p. 134).

> Douglas MacArthur: "There is no security on this earth, there is only opportunity."

As a wealth creator you have to be clear that the choice is never between risk and safety, it is rather a choice between *the kind and degree of risk* that you take. That's because, as Robert Allen says, which is reflected by all of the researchers in this field say, "There is no such thing as financial security." (p. 268).

"With increasing risk, you need increasing levels of courage, and there is no courage without fear, economic or otherwise." (Stanley, 2000, p. 168)

"The risk of failure is always present, but millionaires learn how to deal with economic risk and ultimately keep control of their fears." (Stanley, 2000, p. 135)

"There is a clear and very significant correlation between willingness to take financial risk and net worth." (Stanley, p. 145)

Building your Meta-State of Courage

What components do you need in your context to create the meta-state of courage? There are many ways to build the gestalt state of courage. It all depends on the specific state-on-state arrangement you put together. Here are some possibilities of states to bring to your state of sensing risk to create courage:

Playful risk-taking danger
Joyous excitement of fear (or in spite of fear)
Boldness to take risks in reaching objective
Overwhelming sense of your desired outcome or value
Not-caring for what others say or think while moving forward
Rejecting concern about embarrassment as irrelevant

First, begin by identifying the referent experience in which you want courage to emerge. What wealth building activity, situation, context, etc. would you want or need "courage?"

Where and when and in what context? What for you is fearful about it? What do you find intimidating? What triggers your hesitation?

Now as with any complex meta-stating, flush out your current frames and meta-states about the triggering event or your reactive state.

> What's fearful, threatening, dangerous, etc. about this situation? What do you think-and-feel about your fear? How well does the fear serve you? Do your thoughts-and-feelings about the fear serve you? Have you had enough of this old fear dominating your life? Are you fully ready to reject the old meanings and feelings?

> How did they become millionaires? They saw an economic opportunity that others just ignored and had the willingness to take financial risk.
>
> "There is a strong correlation between one's willingness to take financial risk and one's level of wealth."
> Thomas Stanley

Now you're ready to meta-state the resources to elicit the gestalt state of courage. To do that you might experiment with boldness, passion, compelling outcome, excitement, curiosity, playfulness, etc. Access and bring one resource state at a time and apply to the primary state of fear. Has courage now emerged for you? What else do you need?

When courage emerges from the layering of your meta-stating, then confirm and consolidate it.

> With all of this in mind, how does *this* [fire anchor for the gestalt state] affect this [the referent experience]? How does it transform the situation for you? Do you like this? Are you fully aligned with this? Any objections? Will you keep this? How?

Courage Risk Management
Why aren't more people wealth creators and investors? Kiyosaki answers this question with one word—*risk*. People are afraid of losing. He says that it is a game of skill and that people who turn their money over to someone else to invest are essentially investing in a game they have not learned to play. They are trusting that someone else will play it for them. And that's the problem. *Yet risk can be virtually eliminated—if you know the game.* Managing risk requires knowledge, skills, and a mind-set that you are responsible for yourself.

If there are risk management skills, what are they? And how can you develop them? How can you become open to making mistakes in order to accelerate your learning? What are the skills for learning to take smart risks?

The first thing is to shift your focus from trying to *avoid* risk to effectively *managing* risk. To do that, adjust your thinking by accepting that risk is a part of the game. Accepting that there is no escape from risk allows you to focus on managing it well instead of looking for an imaginary escape. To avoid that, use this mantra: "There is no financial security."

> **The Risk Principle**
> To create wealth you have to take the initiative in discovering trends, markets, making plans, and taking actions. There is no wealth building without some risk. The key is learning how to take *smart* risks.

Once you do that, then begin to learn the game so that you can become skillful in playing it. Intelligently gather information about markets, trends, industry, skills, etc. Critical knowledge will reduce your sense of risk. What area of risk do you need to understand more thoroughly?

Managing risks requires that you take a proactive stance and that your proactively start now with small actions. The very act of taking action will reduce your fear and the sense of risk. As you choose to be self-directed, refuse the negative evaluations of others. As you proactively own your responses— your mental and emotional responses, you build your sense of self-authority and are able to refuse to take counsel of your fears.

Regarding investing, don't wait to save and invest. Start now to save and to invest. Once you have started, continue to do so regularly. About investing, the key is time: "It's a matter of *time* in the market, not the *timing* of the market." As you take a proactive stance, you go on the offense rather than on the defense. Start small. Stop waiting for the big deal and just get into the game now with some small deals.

The amazing thing is that the act of investing money has a way of increasing your intelligence very quickly. Yet to do so, you'll need to refuse to give in to the retarding influence of fear and hesitation. Be willing to initiate. What happens when you experience inertia? Are you willing to push through it? What rituals can you invent to help you move through the deadening feeling of inertia?

The next step in the process of managing risk is to focus on what you can do now. What can you do? What would be even a small first step that would begin to break up the paralyzing nature of fear? At first, buy and hold. Embrace uncertainty and ambiguity and invent it as you go.

> "One of the hallmarks of discipline is one's ability to become economically successful without being given a road map. Millionaires make their own road maps, and no one tells them what time to wake up and go to work." (Stanley, 2000).

One risk-managing step that I really like is to become a futurist. That is, look for large level trends in your particular markets so that you can and distinguish short-term and long-term trends. Then courageously experiment.

> "The only way to innovate: experiment in a chaotic process until a breakthrough occurs." (Dent, 1998, p. 62)

Keep searching for and experimenting with how to create and/or add value. In changing and turbulent economic times, wealth is both being created and transferred. In that case, from where and to where is it being transferred? Do you know? Are you willing to find out? Keep confident in your skills, and abilities in good times and bad times.

As you do all of this make sure you also *take charge of your meanings*. What meanings do you give to things that create fear and risk in the first place? As you commit yourself to facing your fears, explore them, detect their frames, and begin reframing them. What fears hold you back? Is it the fear of losing, the fear of looking foolish, the fear of making a mistake, the fear of attempting something that has no guarantees?

> "The rich don't work for money; money works for them. Don't play it safe, play it smart."
> Kiyosaki (1997)

Another step: Build a security system for yourself and your wealth creation plan. Have you yet created a safety net? Do you have funds available that protect you from getting into trouble with your finances? How much do you need? Why do you need that much? Have you developed a Plan B or Plan C if things go south?

Develop the strength of true security. If there is no security, then what is "true security?" True security is your inner wealth. It is the security you have within—in your mind, strategies, flexibility, learning, friendships, etc. So as you trust your mind, your wits, and your relationship skills to create wealth, you'll develop your self-efficacy. That is, you'll be securing yourself in your knowledge, experience, and abilities.

Finally, do you know your risk level? What is it? This refers to the skill of balancing risk and safety according to your personality and circumstances. So as you know your own risk tolerance, you'll be able to risk at levels where you can stay relaxed and mentally calm. Doing this will take the emotions out of investing and enable you to invest in a more systematic way. Will you need to find an objective financially advisor? That's usually an excellent thing to do.

> *The Smart Risk Principle:* To create wealth you have to take risks, but not risk that threaten your financial welfare, only those that make possible the new opportunities.

> "How much money can you stand to lose? That's how much risk you should assume. If you can't afford to lose it, play it safe. Never fall in love with your investments. Do that and you're in big trouble. To be a visionary and to be a billionaire, you have to chase impossibilities. Few ever get rich easily." (Trump, p. 63)

> "You're fooling yourself to think that you can become financially independent without taking some investment risk." (Stanley, 2000, p. 140)

> "Courage can be developed, but it cannot be nurtured in an environment that eliminates all risks, difficulties and dangers." (Stanley, 171)

Holding a Risky Conversation
If you have never held a conversation about a risk that you are considering, consider finding someone who can ask you the following questions and to do so without giving advice. The power of holding a *risky conversation* is that it gives you a chance to think through the factors and experiences that you feel are risky. Typically, the result is that you will significantly reduce the sense of risk. The key here will be to find someone who will *offer no advice*, who will just ask the questions

and let you find your own answers.

Questions for the Risky Conversation:
1) What is the risk? What is the specific risk?
2) How is it a risk? How do you know? What criteria do you use?
3) What are you risking? (i.e., money, reputation, looking foolish, time)
4) To what extent are you risking this?
5) What is the probabilities of the risk? How much of a risk from 0 to 10?
6) What resources do you have and need to handle the risk?
7) What is the risk now?

The Meta-State of Persistence

Persistence is the sustained effort in pursuing your aims in the face of opposition or difficulty. As such, persistence empowers you to persevere, hang-in, and bounce back from set-backs. Things will happen, challenges will arise, there will be set-backs. Yet if you have incorporated resilience and persistence, you will not be defeated.

> **The Persistence Principle:**
> Wealth is created through persistence, focus on your passion and developing your mastery as you follow your plan for years.

To persist at a task, job, or work you need to let it become absorbing, to find value in it, and to manage your states. The self-made millionaires stayed with their vision and persisted in learning, growing, and becoming more skilled and competent. Tenacity depends on the intensity and purity of your vision which then enables you to stick to your dreams.

Wealth creation is *not* for the weak of heart, but strong, resilient, and dedicated. William Feather writes that "Success seems to be largely a matter of hanging on after others have let go." And W. Clement Stone says, "Every adversity has the seed of an equivalent or greater benefit."

Precisely because persistence is a state of mind based upon definiteness of purpose, desire, self-reliance, definite plans, accurate knowledge, cooperation, and habit, it can be cultivated. You can cultivate it.

Napoleon Hill modeled the secret of wealth accumulation at the request of Dale Carnegie.

"A twenty-year research of hundreds of well-known men, many of whom admitted that they had accumulated their vast fortunes through the aid of the Carnegie secret. (pp. 16-17).

"I had the happy privilege of analyzing both Mr. Edison and Mr. Ford, year by year, over a long period of years and therefore, the opportunity to study them at close range, so I speak from actual knowledge when I say that *I found no quality save persistence,* in either of them, that even remotely suggested the major source of their stupendous achievements. ... persistence, concentration of effort, and definiteness of purpose were the major sources of their achievements." (p. 164)

As Thomas Stanley and William Danko (*1996*) researched those who are wealthy in America, they came up with some *surprising secrets.*

"How do you become wealthy? Here, too, most people have it wrong. It is seldom luck or inheritance or advanced degrees or even intelligence that enables people to amass fortunes. Wealth is more often the result of a lifestyle of hard work, perseverance, planning, and most of all, self-discipline." (pp. 1-2)

Here is a statement that includes a number of elements in a recipe of wealth creation. As you read that as a gestalt meta-state, notice the importance of persistence. Who becomes wealthy?

> "The foundation stones of financial success are *integrity* (being honest with all people), *discipline* (applying self-control), *social skills* (getting along with people), *a supportive spouse*, and *hard work* (more than most people)."
> Thomas Stanley
> *The Millionaire Mind* (p. 11)

"Usually the wealthy individual is a businessman who has lived in the same town for all of his adult life. This person owns a small factory, a chain of stores, or a service company. He has married once and remains married. He lives next door to people with a fraction of his wealth. He is a compulsive saver and investor. He has made his money on his own. Eighty percent of America's millionaires are first-generation rich." (Stanley and Danko, p. 3)

"Those who have cultivated the habit of persistence seem to enjoy insurance against failure. No matter how many times they are defeated, they finally arrive toward the top of the ladder." (Napoleon Hill, p. 154)

Stanley adds this about persistence:

"Most millionaires never allowed poor grades to destroy their goal to succeed. ... *Tenacity* is part of the millionaire's character. Most learn early to fight and compete for important goals" (p. 106)

Machtig speaks about persistence in the overall strategy of wealth creation in these words:
> "Patience and compound interest are two absolutely essential keys to wealth. Successful investors understand that wealth accumulation takes time, so they don't look for short-term bonanzas." (p. 65)

Building the Persistence You'll Need
How do you build a meta-state of persistence? First identify and/or create seemed robust meanings about persistence. What representations, frames, and beliefs stimulate a sense of persistence in you? What are the three most powerful meanings for persistence for you?

Then create your plan for amplifying and integrating your persistence frame. How will you amplify this? How will you integrate this? Will you mind-to-muscle the principle of persistence?

Next you will want to develop a cultural environment to support your persistence. Do you have a cultural environment to support your persistence? What will you do to create the environment that you need? What will you do in your home, office, etc.? Who will hold you accountable to do this? Who will be your coach?

All of your answers to these questions will now enable you to create an action plan for developing persistence. Do you now have an action plan? How strong is your persistence now? What things would undermine or sabotage your persistence? How will you handle those challenges? Are you willing to keep refining this until persistence becomes part of your character and way of being in the world?

Efficiency
Having personal efficiency means allocating your time, energy, and money efficiently and in ways that are most conducive to creating wealth. Stanley and Danko:
> "Efficiency is one of the most important components of wealth accumulation. People who become wealthy allocate their time, energy, and money in ways consistent with enhancing their net worth." (1996, p. 71).

When you are efficient with your time, energy, focus, mind, emotions, etc. you have more of these resources and you get more from them. To become more efficient, begin by first looking for "waste" in your life.
- Where do you waste time, energy, effort, etc.?
- What can you delegate out to others?
- How can you design a more efficient system for your use of time and energy so that you don't have to re-do projects?
- How committed are you to efficiency and to eliminating waste?

The Efficiency Principle: We create wealth through learning to be efficient in your use of energy, time, effort, etc.

Building Efficiency for Your Inside-Out Wealth
Meta-state efficiency by first identifying the context where you need to be more efficient. What do you need to do more efficiently? Where? In what area of your life? How are you *not* efficient in this now?

Next, elicit the feeling of efficiency. Have you ever been efficient? Do you know what that's like? What is the feeling of efficiency for you? Have you ever experienced an activity or series of actions in which for you there was no waste of time, effort, or thought? What is it like for you when you recall that fully? How do you feel when fully in this state? Where? Were you focused, direct, straightforward, moving through activities with ease, in flow? What enabled you to have this experience? What resources made it possible?

Next identify the interferences to efficiency. Are there any interferences for you to become efficient in this activity? Does anything stop you? Do you have full permission? Are there any semantic blocks around such words as "work," "orders," "discipline," etc.?

Check your intention. Why would you want to be efficient here? What's in it for you? What do you get that's of importance? Do you have a big enough why to do what it takes? Will you? Now with all of these resource frames, you are ready to meta-state yourself for efficiency.

> Let's now *feel this* [fire anchor for efficiency] while you think of your context ... and notice how it transforms things... What is that like for you?

Confirm and solidify this state. Do you like this? Can you come up with some supportive frames? Will you? Are you aligned with this?

Resilience
Resilience is a toughness that enables you to bounce back when you are knocked down or when the achievement of your goal is set back. And it is a key meta-state for wealth creation. Kiyoaski wrote this about resilience:
> "Financial freedom has a price. . . . Freedom's price is measured in dreams, desire, and the ability to overcome disappointments that occur to all of us along the way." (p. 46).

I especially like what news commentator, Paul Harvey, wrote about resilience:
> "Someday I hope to enjoy enough of what the world calls success so that someone will ask me, 'What's the secret of it?' I shall say simply this: 'I get up when I fall down.'"

To develop the bounce of resilience requires that you learn how to welcome and handle frustration. If you don't learn to handle frustration, frustration will kill your dreams. Frustration can change a positive attitude into a negative one. One of the worse things that a negative attitude does is wipe out your self-discipline and persistence. When discipline goes, so do the results you desire.

Actually, the key to success is massive frustration. Just look at any person who has achieve any great success. After all, those who are paid some of the highest wages are those who are able to handle the biggest frustrations. The principle is that the more frustration you can handle, the more you can be paid. So aim to learn how to handle frustration effectively. Success is hidden on the inside of frustration.

> **The Resilience Principle:**
> Wealth is built by effectively handling disappointments, frustrations, set-backs, things that are not going right, and bouncing back to your plan and passion.

Transform your old rejection responses. The fear of "No" stops most people from taking action. Learn how to strip "No" of all of its semantic power. Refuse to turn failures into "Big Events!" Do you know how many *"Nos"* can you take? Any *No* has power over you depending on how you give it power through your representations and frames. Why not set an anchor to "No" which turns you on with excitement, determination, and persistence?

To be resilient, identify the resources that put bounce in you. Then take the time to install each one until you have the sense of 'bounce' or resilience within you. So what puts bounce inside you? After you make a list of resources that do that, how will you access and integrate these into your mind and body?[1]

My Personal Story
Of the four meta-states within this chapter, the two that have been the most challenging for me are courage and efficiency. I worked on courage when I decided to launch an attempt of using a media blitz to promote Neuro-Semantics. In 2000 I hired a publicist with the objective to get me onto Oprah's book club. Contact with Harper Productions gave me a set of choices about what would interest Oprah. That led me to decide to create and publish a book on weight management using the Neuro-Semantic approach. As a result, I wrote *Games that Fit and Slim People Play* (2001).

In early 2001 I tested the process with fifteen people. They read the text with the intention of losing weight and attaining a healthy and fit state. And that gave me several people who were ready and able to appear on the program with me. I then signed a contract for ads in *Radio and TV Report,* a nation-wide publication sent twice a month to every radio and television producer. The publication provides the producers information on people who are ready to be interviewed. That cost more than a thousand dollars a month and I signed up for half a year to begin with. The first ad came out in the August edition and during that month I did 52 radio and 3 television interviews. In early September I did another 11 interviews, and then September 11 occurred.

Yes, that brought an end to that. On that day, I received calls from 15 radio stations canceling planned interviews. Suddenly, no one wanted to do a program on weight management. That topic was no longer hot. So the whole process of building up momentum for the national programs was suddenly cut short. And the investment of many thousands failed to achieve what I had hoped.

Although I could have interpreted the whole experience as a failure, I was never even tempted to do that. Rather than a failure, I took it as a learning and a challenge. What enabled me to do that? I was able to take courage from the beginning because I had a clear understanding of the probabilities in taking the risk. The courage was born from knowing that there were no guarantees from the beginning. And of all thing things that I could have anticipated that might have interrupted things, terrorist attacks was not even on my worry list! Consequently, I decided to focus what I learned in the process, the people I met along the way, and the skills I developed. Since I viewed it as an experiment, I did not put a "demand" on it that it had to achieve a certain result.

Your Adventure in Creating Wealth

Okay, time for your Wealth Coaching. Your writing assignment from this chapter is to use your *Wealth Creation Adventure Journal* and to explore the four higher meta-states mentioned in this chapter. How are you doing with the four higher or meta-states of courage, persistence, efficiency, and resilience? Gauge them from 0 to 10 in terms of how much you have each of these states?

Now gauge how rich and robust are your thoughts, ideas, and beliefs which facilitate the access of these states? What are the specific words, beliefs, images, metaphors, etc. that best evoke these powerful states in you? How can you enhance these thoughts to create even more powerful experiences of these states? What practices will you begin to give yourself to this week that will develop and/or strengthen these states?

End of Chapter Notes

1. My original research on resilience (1991-1994) resulted in the discovery of the Meta-States Model. In the book *Meta-States* (2008) I tell that story as well as included a chapter on Resilience. For more about resilience, we have as training manual, "Resilience: The Ability to Bounce Back."

Chapter 13

CAN I HAVE FUN DOING ALL OF THIS?

"You have to love what you're doing, because then it won't seem like work to you and you will bring the necessary energy to profit from it. That *passion* alone will take care of ninety percent of any problems with any job."

Donald Trump

In the past two chapters we have examined a great many wealth creation states. In chapter 11 we looked the general process of accessing states and meta-stating higher states to create complex gestalt states. I also described the process for how to release sabotaging states. In chapter 12 you examined four critical meta-states that are essential for wealth creation, namely, courage, persistence, efficiency, and resilience.

If in all of that, you didn't choose some *joyful states,* the time has now come to do that. After all, creating wealth should be a lot of fun, shouldn't it? And if you have developed the inner wealth of choosing, accessing, and experiencing the states that you want, then you have the *being* and *doing* wealth of state creation. So the question I am posing in this chapter is this:

> How can you become *playfully rich* as you engage in wealth creation? How can you have *lots of fun* so that the intensity of the engagement will be delightful for you and others?

I have designed this chapter to present the answer to these questions as *seven steps for becoming playfully rich*. This is critically important because one of the central wealth creation secrets that the researchers found is the power of engagement in something that they found that the self-made millionaires believed in and enjoyed. *Enjoyed*—they got a kick out of doing something which they found fascinating and absorbing. That is, *they had fun in the process*. They believed that life is good and rich with things worthwhile and things to enjoy and they did not want to miss it. If that's a secret for inside-out wealth, then how can you access and experience that secret?

> **The Playful / Fun Principle:**
> We create wealth by staying light and playful rather than serious. Wealth is created by transforming our work as a source of enjoyment.

1) Refuse to dichotomize work and play.
Whenever you think about "work," be sure to connect it to fun, joy, and play. Don't dichotomize these two experiences. Don't separate them as if they are opposites. If you dichotomize work and play, you will then be constantly looking for how to get out of work or how to work minimally. And that very orientation will undermine your ability to create quality products and services that add value to others. Do the opposite: give work your very best in your work and turn it into fun.

The fact is, you will become more productive when you turn your work a joy. Yet only a minority of workers today absolutely love their work. One secret of the successful is that they feel compelled in their passion, they give themselves to it long enough to become highly competent and they seldom think of it as "work." They think of it as play or a wonderful privilege. The ability to enjoy your work gives you a real source of wealth. So as you learn to see your "work" in terms of play, you won't fall into the pit of dichotomizing your work from your play.[1]
   Abraham Maslow (1954) spoke to this a long time ago:
> "At the highest level of living, i.e., of Being, duty *is* pleasure, one's 'work' is loved, and there is no difference between working and vacationing." (1970 edition, p. 102).

2) Turn your work into play.
It's not enough to *not* dichotomize, you also have to *positively*

transform your work so that it feels like play. As you stop separating work and play, the next question is how to combine the two. How can you enjoy your work? How can you make the whole process of creating wealth fun and enjoyable? How can you structure it, and your attitude towards it, so that you experience it as a reward? How can you transform it from drudgery work into a life-style that you will find as challenging as it is compelling?

The answers is to return to the essence of wealth—*valuing and the state of appreciating, enjoying, and delighting.* If you know this, you can then frame all of the wealth creating activities with a spirit of joy. Do that and you make the process fun and rewarding in and of itself. To transform your work and effort into a form of enjoyment and delight, plant the appreciation question into your mind: *What can I appreciate about my work?* What can I appreciate about the effort that's required? How can I incorporate a playful spirit into all of the things that I do?

> "Work as hard as thou canst. If he does not appreciate all thou do, never mind. Work well-done, does good to the man who does it. It makes him a better man." (Clawson, *The Richest Man in Babylon*, p 124).

3) Change your attitude about the effort of work.

If you find step two difficult, it may be because you need a change of attitude. So, do you know how to turn work into fun? "Work" will become the best friend you've ever known for creating wealth if you treat it as a friend. If your attitude is, "Only slaves work," then you obviously will defeat yourself with that belief frame. If you believe, "Wealth will free me from even needing to work or expending effort," that belief also itself will prevent you from using your work as a source of wealth. Nor will you get ahead by shirking.

So, what's your attitude about work? When you hear the word "work," what is the first thing that comes to mind? How do you represent it in your head— what are the pictures and sounds in your mind about it? And when you think about what you do for a living, does the word "work" seem to fit?

I best like to think of *work* as a child thinks about play. If you have never really watched children play, you'll notice that it involves a lot of effort. They expend a lot of energy in playing! They run, jump, yell, twist, pull, push and so on in a fury of actions that involves an incredible amount of effort and energy. Yet it isn't work for them, it is play. It is fun. Even when I was a young parent— keeping up with a bunch of children seemed like a lot of work! And often it was for me, but not for them. Now what if you exerted that level of energy and effort into what you otherwise would call your "work?"[2]

4) Learn to love your job.
Because love, fun, and joy all go together, *the more love you put into things, the more fun you will have.* The more you invest your work with love, the more you'll be able to enjoy it. So develop a love for what you do, the contributions you make, and the difference you make. And love it so much that it feels like you are on vacation every day. This is what Donald Trump thinks and feels:

> "Don't take vacations. What's the point? If you're not enjoying your work, you're in the wrong job. We do it because it's fun. Work hard, play hard, and live to the hilt. Be under-estimated. It's more impressive if people discover your accomplishments without you telling them. Impress people through results. Billionaires love their jobs. You have to love what you're doing, because then it won't seem like work to you and you will bring the necessary energy to profit from it. That *passion* alone will take care of ninety percent of any problems with any job." (2004, p. 81).

Kioysaki goes even further. He even calls wealth creating *a game,* "It's only a game" he says repeatedly. Then he compares the whole thing to the game of Monopoly.

> "Life really is a game of *monopoly* for people on the right side of the quadrant. Sure, there is winning and losing, but that is part of the game. Winning and losing is a part of life. To be successful on the right side of the quadrant is to be a person who *loves the Game.*" (p. 154)

And what's to be loved? If you don't know, then return to chapter 3 and use the intentionality pattern repeatedly until you find your *big why*. Your big why will be your "happy thoughts" that, like Peter Pan, will enable you to fly.

5) Transform work into an experience of vitality.
While you can make lots of money without physical or personality health, the lack of health in these two dimensions will not allow you to experience fullness, authenticity, joy, and pleasure. This is a key reason for cultivating your inner vitality. Unhealthy attitudes and beliefs can

undermine the expression of working to create financial wealth and sabotage your experience of the richness of life.

So what is your relationship to your work and effort? Do you feel more alive at the end of the day than at the beginning? Have you developed the skills for taking pleasure, satisfaction, and delight in doing a good job? What resources do you need in order to do that? *Anything—and everything—can become a pleasure in human experience.* Even handling grumpy customers, could become a source of satisfaction, and even delight, when well done if you have the right attitude.

This mental vitality also depends on physically feeling well and energetic. And that relates to how you are taking care of yourself and exercising regularly. Stanley (2000) writes about this when he says:
> "Keeping in excellent physical condition can be an important tool in dealing with detractors because it helps to one's competitive spirit." (p. 51)
> "Fatigue brings out the worst in people who are confronted with job-related stress and financial risk." (p. 171)

Do you have the vitality that comes from having a healthy and fit body? Do you watch your eating, exercising, stretching, relaxing to develop a relaxed and clear mind? These are the elements that will increase your sense of personal aliveness. What belief frame would you need to keep you focused on sound physical health? Find it and integrate it.

6) *Discover how to use wealth shaping.*
From the field of Behavioral psychology (or Learning Theory) comes the whole idea of shaping or conditioning. The basic principle is to use reinforcements to reward whatever you want to become a habit in your actions. What will you use? It depends on what you find reinforcing. When you find something rewarding, use it to shape the actions you want to turn into a habit.

As you can shape the responses in animals and in people, you can also shape the responses that will empower you to succeed in creating the life you want. This means that you can shape your own behaviors, attitudes, emotions, skills, responses, etc.

To use reinforcement shaping, make a list of ten or fifteen activities that cost nothing, or very little, and yet which you highly value and have a lot of fun doing. List activities that gives you a sense of vitality, energy, renewed power, love, courage, orderliness, health, etc. Make a list of these behaviors. Don't limit your list to just pure pleasures, think in terms of rejuvenation and the renewing of your visions.

> **The Vitality Principle**:
> It takes energy and effort to create value and to build wealth and so staying healthy and fit is essential and part of internal physical wealth—the sense of physical vitality.

   1) Pure pleasures
   2) Rejuvenating activities

When you complete this, you have created a list of activities that you find personally and uniquely rewarding. You now have in your hands a tool for adding massive pleasure to your life. Now you can consciously and intentionally reward yourself with one or more of these highly valued rewarding activities every time you take another step in the direction that supports your wealth creation plans. The design is to reward yourself with value-rich activities that give you a sense of pleasure and fun. You will be able to distinguish between mere indulgences and true pleasures.

I learned to do this with the task of categorizing my receipts at the end of the year and prepare them for my accountant. Once that task started taking a lot of time (more than three hours), I developed a ritual. Sometime at the first of January each year, I set aside half a day for it. I put on some classic music, set out a glass of wine, and then pull out my boxes of receipts. I do the ones for the publishing company; then for the investment properties; then for the training business.

January in Colorado is typically cold and snowy; so it's a really nice time to be inside. I put on a fire in the fireplace, stretch out the receipts on a table and begin categorizing and recording the amounts spent in various areas. The first time I created and used this ritual, it felt very strange—weird in fact. But as the Januarys have come and gone, I now look forward to the ritual— as a time for taking care of business.

7) *Enjoy generously giving back.*

Having lots of money can mean many things. Among these one thing that it can mean is that you can give back to people you love and causes you believe in. After all, why make money? What will you spend it on? Who will you spend it on? Only on you? Who else would you like to bless?

> **The Abundance Principle:**
> We build wealth by operating from abundance, believing in abundance, acting with abundance, and cultivating abundance.

And when will you do this? The fact is you don't have to wait until you have millions, you can begin to experience the joy, and the state of being, a benefactor. Anthony Robbins recommend dividing your income into a 10/10/10/70 proportion. This means— live on 70 percent of what you have, save 10% to build up capital to invest, reduce all debts with another 10%, and give away another 10% of your income.

> "The secret of living is giving. Give first. If you're just accumulating money for you, to lord it over your kingdom, you are not really a success, don't really have power, nor true wealth. Think of success as *a process, a way of life,* and a strategy for living. Then use your power in a responsible and loving way. Re-invest money regularly as an expression of your mission to make the world a better place and to make yourself the master of money, not its slave." (*Unlimited Power*, 1988)

There's another benefit in learning how to give back. You will discover how to extend yourself to others. And that's important. That will enable you to get out of yourself, get your ego out of the way. After all, adding value to others is the central process for creating wealth. So wealth creation from the beginning to the end is never about you. And all of this will enable you to act from the position of abundance thereby making you a more generous as a person. Giving back also provides a great context for learning what money can do and what it cannot do.

What is the psychology within the experience of giving freely to endow a person or a cause? Psychologically it communicates the idea of abundance—that you have plenty, that the sources of wealth are abundant, and that there is no scarcity.

My Personal Story

While I have lots of fun studying, discovering new things, articulating life-changing ideas, and then creatively packaging in ways for people to use, I often get so caught up in the process that it seems like work to those who are watching from the outside. "You sure are working hard!" people comment to me as they greet me when I'm at coffee at Starbucks in the morning. The comment sometimes interrupts me from the experience of being lost in the moment, "What?" I ask. "You're always reading, don't you ever do something for fun?"

I hardly know how to answer that question. *I am having fun!* Probably not their fun, but certainly my fun. And the effort I expand in my studies is a good bit of the fun. And why would I go and do something else, something different, to get away from the fun I'm having? "What do you do just for fun?" a former attorney asked me recently at Starbucks. "Why this!" I said nodding to the book I was reading and to the notes I was making. Then after a long pause, he added, "Anything else?"

The most fun part of the real estate for me is the adventure of finding a new investment. Knowing that the profit is made at the purchase rather than at the sale, I love the exploration. It's like hunting for treasure. I also get a big kick out of taking a sorely mistreated house and nursing it back to health. I like the remodeling, painting, improving, and seeing a house and yard become functional and attractive—a place to grow a family.

The part I didn't like at first was being called upon or informed about problems with the house. You know, being called about things that need fixing—toilets, air conditioners, kitchen appliances. At first I experienced that as a hassle and an irritation. Then year after year, as I would do the year-end analysis, recording the expenses for a house, I found myself in a different state —not in the state of wanting to save money, or not spend money on repairs. I would rather be in a state of looking for all of the expenses I could find and deduct which I spent on repairs. And if there was not sufficient expenses to deduct on my taxes, I'd experience a disappointment. "I didn't spend much on that property this year." "I need to do better next year." Eventually I was able to access this perceptual state when someone call about repairs. And when I was able to do that, my response changed to, "Great!"

Your Adventure in Creating Wealth

As your Wealth Coach, what will you choose as your key activities that you will use to integrate into your *fun wealth activities*? To discover such, first make a list of the fun states that you experience as part of your way of creating wealth.

- Now gauge the level of fun that you have in these states. From 0 to 10, how much fun do you have?
- What can you appreciate about your work? Make a list of ten things.
- How will you increase your sense of joyful fun in creating wealth? How can you turn up your fun so that it increases to a high level?
- What set of actions will you take in order to tap into this source of inner wealth?

As you step back from the seven steps for becoming playfully rich, which of these have you already achieved and which are the ones yet to be developed?

1) Refuse to dichotomize work and play.
2) Turn your work into play.
3) Change your attitude about the effort of work.
4) Learn to love your work.
5) Transform work into an experience of vitality.
6) Discover how to use wealth shaping.
7) Enjoy generously giving back.

End of Chapter Notes

1. About the joy of being fully engaged, see the chapter in *Unleashing Leadership* (2009) on engagement.

2. Beliefs create attitudes so if you need to change an attitude, find and change the beliefs that form and govern the attitude. This is a meta-state process. See *Winning the Inner Game* (2007) for the belief change process.

Chapter 14

WHAT ARE THE PRINCIPLES OF WEALTH CREATION?

Most books about wealth creation are written at the level of principles. They state great ideas, conceptual understandings, and rules about how wealth is created. The value of knowing these principles is that they inspire a general understanding. There's also a problem with this approach. The ideas are presented so generally that they do not give you a specific blueprint for how to create wealth. While they may present *the what*, they leave you on your own to figure out the *how-to*.

Principles about wealth creation are generally written as the basic "factors," "secrets," "rules," and "steps." Most principles are stated as universals and often sound like truisms or Ancient Chinese philosophy. These principles are the great ideas for how to play the great game of wealth creation. Principles articulate a general map for navigating a particular dimension of life.

When I first began reading in the area of finances, wealth creation, and economic success, many of these wonderful principles jumped out and caught my attention. "That's a fabulous idea!" I then had a second thought, "So what am I supposed to do to make use of that great idea?" I found this especially frustrating. And out of that frustration eventually emerged a solution—*the Mind-to-Muscle Pattern*. This pattern emerged one day as I was exploring *how* to transfer a mental understanding into a neurological response for how to actualize the idea.

The Mind-to-Muscle pattern enables you to take a conceptual learning that you *know intellectually* and turn it into a something that you *know experientially*. And when you know it experientially, it governs how you live, how you move through the world, how you feel, and how you *live* the information that you know intellectually.

The Mind-to-Muscle pattern is also a meta-stating pattern and its design is to enable you to turn highly informative, insightful, and valued conceptual principles into neurological patterns in your body. If you have learned how to type on a keyboard you have already done this. The original learning may take a considerable amount of time and trouble in order to get the muscle patterns and coordination deeply imprinted into your muscles. Yet by practicing and training, the learnings eventually become incorporated into the very fabric of the muscles. You then lose conscious awareness of the learnings as the muscles can then perform the program. At that point, you have translated principle into muscle.

The same holds true for expertise, excellence, and mastery in all other fields, from sports, mathematics, teaching, to surgery, selling, and public relations. Begin with a *principle*—a concept, understanding, awareness, belief, etc., and translate it into a neurological pattern in your muscles. I have found this especially true in our modeling projects regarding resilience, leadership, wealth creation, selling excellence, learning, etc. This pattern creates transformation by moving up and down the various levels of mind so that you map from your understandings about something from the lowest descriptive levels to the highest conceptual levels and back down again.

When you learn the pattern, you'll be able to take any great principle about wealth creation and then *coach your body how to feel that principle*. Doing this will *somatize* the concept. There is one warning I need to make about this: Make sure you pick a principle that's true and reliable. The ecology of this pattern is not in the pattern, but in your initial choice. So be sure to pick a good one.

What follows are lots of the general principles for creating wealth that you have encountered in the previous chapters. If you're going to play the Wealth Creation Game, you need to know the rules of the game. So here they ae. Most of obvious; some are not. Take those that will make a transformative difference in your life and use the Mind-to-Muscle pattern at the end of this chapter and integrate them into your way of moving through the world as you see ways to add value and create wealth.

Principles for Creating Wealth about Yourself

Inside-Out Wealth: Wealth is created from the inside out. First create wealth inside, and then design a plan for letting it out into the world via your talents, strengths, passions, and skills.

State of Mind: Wealth is created through a rich creative mind that cares and can translate great ideas into everyday reality.

Creativity: Wealth is created via developing your creative abilities. Wealth arises as you create new valuable solutions to problems.

Self-Discipline: Wealth is created through hard work and self-discipline, through owning your powers and responses and developing them. It takes ownership, responsibility, and accountability to create wealth.

The Right State: Wealth is created from being in the right state. Like everything else in life, if you want to succeed in a particular field, you have to access and operate out of the right state.

Integrity: Wealth is created by developing character, integrity, and the power of congruency.

Decisiveness: Wealth is created through the ability to weigh alternatives, make an informed decision, and stay with it. Wealth is created through making decisions, becoming decisive, and making decisions to stay with our decisions.

Courage: Wealth is created by courage. Creating wealth involves taking risks—smart risks that do not threaten your financial welfare, but those that make possible the new opportunities.

Vitality: Wealth is created by expending energy and effort to create value. Build wealth by staying healthy and fit so you have the physical wealth, a sense of physical vitality.

Fun: Wealth is created by being playful and staying light rather than serious. If you get serious, you will get stupid. Then you will experience a poverty of spirit.

Frugality: Wealth is created by using the delight of frugality in the early stages as you raise your joy-to-stuff ratio and squeeze all the juice out of the things you already have.

Efficiency: Wealth is created by learning to be more efficient in your use of energy, time, and efforts. Wealth is efficiency.

Principles about the Structure and Process of Creating Wealth
Adding Value: Wealth is created by valuing, creating value, and adding value. Wealth in any culture is what we say is valuable, so wealth creation is adding value as we play to our talents and strengths.

Modeling: Wealth is created by modeling good examples of people who have created wealth in a way that maintains their integrity, values, and relationships.

Communication: Wealth is created by working with and through people which necessitates clear and compelling communication for understanding, rapport, and negotiations. Wealth is rich collaborative partnerships.

Collaboration: Wealth is created through cooperating with others, networking, finding mentors, being mentors, etc. Wealth is built by effectively working with and through others.

Networking: Wealth is created by networking. You do better in any domain of effort within which you seek to achieve excellence when you have like-minded and supportive others on your team. Social support emerges when men and women of like mind, get together for networking, brainstorming, encouragement, accountability, etc.

Seeing Opportunities: Wealth is created by seeing and seizing opportunities to solve problems and add value.

Solving Problems: Wealth is created by a love of hunting to find and solve problems. People pay best for solutions to their most serious and important problems.
Money: Wealth is created by de-loading the semantic load on "money."

Wealth is *not* money. Wealth is created by separating it from status, person, identity, etc. Do that and you become free to become truly wealthy. Wealth is *not* money. Money is a sign or a scoreboard of wealth.

Financial Wisdom: Wealth is created when you recognizing that money is important. Money is crucial for financial freedom so that it works for you without making you its slave.

Selling and Negotiating: Wealth is created by selling yourself, your ideas, your products, and your services. Wealth is created via promoting and selling the value that you offer. You have to get the word out about that.

Initiative: Wealth is created by taking the initiative in discovering trends, markets, making plans, and taking actions. There's no wealth building without some risk.

Persistence: Wealth is created over time through patience and persistence.

Resilience: Wealth is created through effectively handling disappointments, frustrations, set-backs, things not going right, and bouncing back to your plan and passion.

Meta-Detailing: Wealth is created by detailing out the specifics of your business from a meta-position. Synthesizing global and specific enables you to know where you are and take care of the killer details.

Principles about Talent by which we Create Wealth

Planning: Wealth is created by developing a plan for how to manage finances, focus attention on skills, interests, passions, and talents in adding value.

Entrepreneurship: Wealth is created by adopting the attitudes and mind-set of an entrepreneur who assumes complete responsibility for his or her own financial independence.

Focus: Wealth is created at first through concentration. Concentrate on your inner wealth and talent first; diversify in the latter steps.

Principles about Money and Finances for Wisdom

Financial Intelligence: Wealth is created by developing the financial intelligence to understand how to handle money and use it as an effective tool.

Income: Financial independence is created through increasing income, developing multiple sources of income, and inventing systems for passive income. It is created by developing enough passive income to exceed expenses.

Savings: Wealth is created by saving. Wealth is about net worth, not income. It's about how much you save, not how high you live.

Managing Money: Wealth is created by effectively managing money—tracking it, budgeting, saving, investing, giving, and enjoying it.

Debts: Wealth is created by getting rid of debts and only accept those that are true investments.

True Assets: Wealth is created by distinguishing investments and liabilities and investing in true assets that increase with value over time.

Taxes: Wealth is created by taking control over your cashflow and savings as you use your financial intelligence to reduce your taxes in every way you can.

Mental Accounting: Wealth is created by clear thinking about money. "A dollar here, a dollar there; pretty soon we're talking about real money." Know the Neuro-Semantics of mental accounting. How you represent, reckon, and appraise "money" determines how you respond to it.

Charging: Wealth is created best by getting paid for results. Value-based fees is entirely performance based.

Passive Income: Financial independence is created through creating sources of passive income. It's created through having passive income that exceeds your expenses.

Money: Wealth is created by valuing money. Money is important for creating the freedom to spend your time and energy on what you care about rather than worrying about paying bills. Money is un-important in the areas in which it cannot work —creating security, love, happiness, creativity, etc.

Spending: Wealth is created by spending less than you make.

Income sources: Wealth is created by increasing the sources of your income, by developing multiple sources of income, and making more than you spend.

Getting Ourselves To Take Action

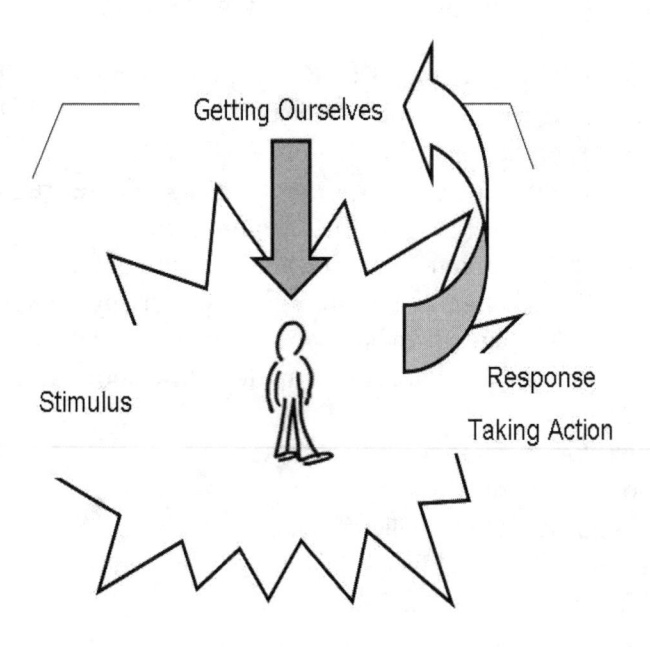

Getting Ourselves

Stimulus

Response

Taking Action

MIND-TO-MUSCLE
Closing the Knowing-Doing Gap Pattern

I have taken the following Mind-to-Muscle pattern straight out of the training manual. It is written there for one person to facilitate it with another. And that is the best way to learn it. Invite someone to read the questions and run the processes so that you can *coach your body to feel and neurologically know* the principle.

The Pattern:
1) Identify a principle or concept you want incorporated in your body.
> What concept or principle do you want to put into your neurology?
> What is your conceptual understanding of this idea?
> What do you know or understand about this that you want to set as a frame in your mind?
> How can you state it in the a way that's clear, succinct, and compelling?
> Finish this sentence stem: *"I understand . . ."*

When you facilitate this or do it with yourself, watch for the natural gestures that you use when you say the words, "I understand that wealth is created by spending less than you make." Note your tone of voice, your muscle tension, your face, your movements. These are expressions of how you operate from the mental conceptual state of an "understanding." It is generally a very weak state in terms of energy in your body. When I am in this state, I gesture with my right hand to my forehead, "I understand..." and my voice is matter-of-fact, calm, and the feel is one of being in an intellectual mode. How about you?

2) Describe the principle as a belief.
> Do you believe this principle?
> Would you like to believe that?
> If you really, really believed that, would that make a big difference in your life?
> State the concept as a belief and notice what happens: *"I believe . . ."*
> Did you state it as if you really believed it?
> As you state it with as much conviction as possible, what do you feel?

In this second step you will be using more of your neurology to say the statement as a belief statement. Again, notice with an exactness the quality of the voice, muscle tension, posture, movements, gestures, face, eyes, etc. as you (or another) says, "I believe that I can create wealth and build capital by spending less than I make." If there is little difference between step 1 and step 2, then return to step 1 and notice your *understanding state* then move into the *belief state* and exaggerate it. If you have to move back and forth several times to notice more and more differences, do so.

When I move into a belief state my gesture completely changes. I now use my right hand moving it in an up-and-down movement, usually with a fist. The muscles in my arm and forearm becomes firm and tense and I speak as if I'm punching the air with my belief statements. My body also tenses up, my breathing becomes stronger, I focus my eyes as I look forward. How about you?

Notice also the linguistic changes that occur. Your statement in step 1 will be intellectual, conceptual, and mental. "Intellectually I understand that wealth is created by adding value by solving the problems and desires of others." When you move to the belief state, the words you say will become more personal and intimate. Now use the personal pronoun words. "I believe that *I* can create wealth by adding value by finding ways that *I* can solve problems for others." How are you feeling as you make your belief statement? What emotions are emerging? Notice those.

3) *Reformat the belief as a decision.*
Would you like to live by that belief? [Yes.] You would? [Yes.] Really? [Yes.]
Will you act on this and make it your program for acting?
State it as a decision saying, *"I will . . ."* *"I want . . . it is time to..."* *I choose to . . ."*
"From this day forward I will .... because I believe..."

From the *belief state* you now move to the *decision state*. Again, it requires more of your neurology to move here and make statements that reflect a decision. I like raising my right hand as if taking a vow. "I will look for ways to add value to people and solve more important problems and so create wealth." "From this day forward, I will spend less than I make."

You will undoubtedly also notice more changes in your body as you move into the *decision state*. My right hand typically gestures to an imaginary line right in front of me and at my feet or a point as if that is the "decision point." And while the tension may be similar to the belief state, the muscles in my forearm and arm moves as if cutting a line. How about you?\

Notice also how your linguistics change. As you keep repeating the belief and decision statements, you are essentially looking for the right words, the best words that summarize your belief and/or decision. "From now on I am going to look for how I can add value and stop looking first for what is in it for me."

How are you feeling as you make your decision statement? What emotions are emerging? Notice those.

4) *State the decision as an emotional state or experience.*
>As you state the belief decision, noticing what you feel, what do you feel?
>What do you feel as you imagine living your life with this empowering belief and decision?
>Be with those emotions . . . let them grow and extend.
>State feelings, *"I feel . . . I experience . . . because I will . . . because I believe . . ."*

Now throughout the two previous steps of belief and decision, feelings, sensations, and emotions will be evoked and rushing through you. Now it's time to use those emotions. Emotions are designed to create *movement* and *motion*. Emotions *move* us to take action and to move out from where we are. So step into the *emotion state* and notice what's happening in your body as you make the statements that increasingly translate the principle into your body.

5) *Turn the emotions into actions.*
>What one thing will you do tomorrow that will begin to manifest this in your life? And the day after that?
>*"The one thing that I will do today to make this real in my life is . . ."*

Now you are ready to use the energy of your emotions, to translate what you feel into what you will do. As you imagine acting on your feelings that the beliefs and decisions elicit from within you, step forward as if you are *doing* something. Also think of actions that are small and simple— telling someone, writing something down, buying a blank book for your business plan, set your clock 15 minutes earlier, etc. What you do is not as important as you *do something*. The whole purpose here is to activate your body and to begin to actually *live* the principle.

6) Step into the action and synergize with the higher levels.

As you fully imagine doing one thing and then another and carrying out what you are going to do to make the principle real in your life . . . seeing, hearing and feeling those actions, just be aware of your answers as I ask them. There's no need to speak aloud, just answer it within yourself. You are doing this because you believe what? Because you've decided what? Because you feel what? And you will do what other thing? Because you understand what? Because you feel what? Because you've decided what? Because you believe what? And what other thing will you do?

And do you like this? Really? Will this make a difference in your life? Will it begin to launch your wealth creation plan? Are you fully aligned with this? Is there anything in the back of your mind that objects to this? So you will keep thi

My Personal Story

I discovered the Mind-to-Muscle pattern originally while preparing for the Wealth Creation training in northern England in 1996. After reading one morning, I felt excited about a particular principle, and I sat back from the table at the coffee shop and reflected. "Intellectually, do I know that?" Yes! I certainly do. Then under my breath I said to myself:

"Intellectually I know that wealth is a human construct and that it can be invented by anyone. That there's an infinite amount of wealth to be created."

Smiling and delighted with that fabulous insight, I then had a second thought, an upsetting one, one that disturbed my peace of mind, and served as a reality check. "But do I believe it? Really? If you believe it, why aren't you experiencing it?" Hmmmm. I was doing provocative coaching with myself and it was creating an immense disequilibrium in my emotions.

"Do I believe it?" Hmmmm. Then again, under my voice I uttered a belief statement,

> "I believe that I can tap into the infinite amount of wealth that is yet to be created and that I can become wealthy."

Now if you had heard my voice, you would have gone, "Yeah, really!" in a tone of skepticism and disbelief. You would have provocatively challenged me, "You really sound like you believe that!"

That's what I heard in myself and I suppose being in a mood of provocation, I challenged myself again. "Okay, say it as if you did believe it!" So I did. Again and again I repeated the statement *as if* I really did believe it and that's when I noticed something. My neurology, my physiology, and my movements and gestures were very different as I stated it as a strong belief. *It took more physiology to make that statement.* It was no longer just an intellectual statement. To a much greater extent, it was a full body experience.

I didn't stop there. My next thought was, "Okay, if I did turn this fabulous idea into a belief, will I actually act on it? I guess I need to make up my mind and make a decision to do it." So I then stated it as a decision:

> "From this day forward I will tap into the infinite amount of wealth that can be created. I will learn how to create wealth, what creates it, and begin to really enrich my wealth creation ten-year plan!"

Talk about a statement that evoked some emotions, that one did! Suddenly, I felt a strong rush of both excitement and fear. Excitement about the possibilities and fear about my actual ability to do that. And there were emotions of ambiguity, doubt, curiosity, and playfulness. I could hardly contained myself at the table and as the energy from all of those emotions rushed through me I stood up, left my books and walked out to the front of the coffee shop. I needed to move. And as I did I wondered, "What can I do today to make this real? This is great; I don't want it to just evaporate or dissipate, how can I plug this into some action and actualize it?"

As I thought of a couple of actions, writing it down, telling someone about it, etc., I remembered what William James wrote about emotions and how that if we use our emotions, take actions on them, we reinforce them and give them real-life expressions. And that's how the Mind-to-Muscle pattern arose.

Since then I have used the pattern hundreds if not thousands of times to translate "knowledge" into procedural knowledge and localize it in my neurology. I best like to do it when I'm exercising because my body is already activated.

Your Adventure in Creating Wealth
For your Wealth Coaching this week, read through the principles in this chapter and identify which one will have the most transformative difference in your life. Run that pattern through the Mind-to-Muscle pattern right now. Repeat five to seven times or until you have the sense of "Of course!" when you first think about the principle.

Next, plan to run one principle each day for the next month. Because the Mind-to-Muscle pattern essentially enables you to commission your body to *know* and to *feel* the principle, be sure you have chosen highly ecological principles.

Chapter 15

DEVELOPING YOUR WEALTH CREATION PLAN

If you want to create wealth, inside-out wealth, then you need a plan. You need a well-developed blueprint or roadmap so that you can get there. Do you remember *the planning questions*?

Do you have a plan? Do you know how to develop a plan? Do you know how to keep refining your plan? Do you know how to follow your plan? Do you know how to keep motivating yourself to pursue your plan?

The Matrix Model provides a way to sort out the facets of wealth creation. The Matrix refers to your layers of mental maps (beliefs, understandings, decisions, etc.) that you have about wealth. It is about what you think and feel about money, work, abundance, budgeting, saving, and much more. This leads to all of your strategies about work, career, education, learning, contribution, creativity, finances, saving, investing, being an entrepreneur, financial independence, etc.
- How do self-made first-generation millionaire's create the wealth that they do?
- What models do we have of their strategies?
- How do self-made first-generation millionaire's think?
- Do you think like a millionaire? To what extend do you, to what extent do you not?

Because your frames control your games, the adventure begins by detecting and identifying your frames. It continues as you then change those that are not serving you well. As you use the Matrix Model, you can create a new inner game. And winning the inner game makes playing the outer game a cinch.

There is a *strategy* for creating wealth to become financially independent. There are thousands of people who are first-generation rich around the world. *How* is it that they are able to do that? Luck? Wealth genes? Superior intelligence? Secret skills? No. *They have discovered the heart of wealth creation.* And they have built a Wealth Matrix that support their ability to create wealth. They build wealth through a very definite set of steps and stages from finding a passion, caring about something, adding value, and finding a way to communicate it effectively.

> "Anyone can wish for riches, and most people do, but only a few know that a definite plan, plus a burning desire for wealth, are the only dependable means of accumulating wealth."
> Napoleon Hill

Inside-out wealth is not built overnight, but over time. Because it arises as you become wealthy *inside,* your success depends on being able to transfer your wealth of ideas, creativity, and value *outside.* In doing that, in a given market, you become more and more valued. Add the required business intelligence to this and financial wealth will follow. Do that and you will discover the true secrets for building wealth that's truly satisfying, invigorating, holistic, and enduring. Sure some win a lottery, or happen upon a source of almost instantaneous wealth, but they are the exceptions, and if they are not ready for wealth, then like most lottery winners, they will not be able to sustain it.

Inside-Out Wealth focuses on the inner game of wealth creation so that you first empower yourself with the necessary frames. This makes creating the outside wealth easy. Your wealth creation lifestyle will then fit your passions, talents, and circumstances. Are you ready to create your own Ten-Year Plan and to develop a business plan of specific actions that you can do each day?

This process will ask you to set many specific goals that establish your direction. It will enable you to actualize your highest and best into your performance. You will incorporate the principles of the game into your mind-body system as beliefs, decisions, states, intentions, pleasures, skills, emotions, and actions.

As you prepare yourself now for wealth . . . know that you will be challenged again and again about the principles and meanings of wealth creation . . . that you will have to fight and tame and even slay some dragons along the way ... that you will be invited to rise up to the highest levels of your mind to adjust your frames, deframe those that get in the way, reframe, and set entirely new frames of meaning and mind ... that you will learn a set of new tools for governing your mind-body system of thoughts, feelings, speech, and behavior. ... and that in the end, you will begin a new journey toward wealth in a holistic way that will enrich your life in many, many ways.

YOUR PERSONALIZED INSIDE-OUT WEALTH CREATION PLAN

What have you learned, or are you learning, about creating your own personalized Wealth Matrix? How robust are your frames of meaning and frames of mind about wealth and these facets of wealth?

In the following pages you have an opportunity to create your very own *Wealth Creation Plan*. As you identify the key variables for inside-out wealth, you create a way to make your plan real in your everyday actions. Fill in these pages and keep refining them until you create a workable plan. As you keep developing your plan, you may wan to transfer it to a computer file. Then you can create a workable blueprint that you can keep refining year by year. If you keep renewing and transforming your plan, it will become more elegant, exquisite, and focused as a wealth creator.

The World Matrix
- What world will you work in to create wealth?
- What financial intelligence do you already have for this area and what financial intelligence will you need to develop?
- What business acumen is required to succeed in this area?

The *Worlds* or domains in which I will create wealth in are —

_____
_____
_____

The *Worlds* that I will learn to navigate for creating wealth include—

_____
_____
_____
_____

The Time Matrix
- What stage of wealth creation are you at right now?
- Do you have a wealth of time?
- What are your next steps in your plan?
- How long will it take? What resources will you need to handle the patience and persistence required?

The meanings, beliefs, and meta-states that best enhance my sense and use of time in creating wealth includes —

_____
_____
_____
_____

My time schedule for creating wealth include the following steps—

_____
_____
_____
_____

The Meaning Matrix
- What is wealth? What does wealth mean to you?
- Do you have a compelling definition of wealth that you find exciting and attractive?

The *meanings* that I am creating about wealth, money, financial independence, etc. which inspire my passions are—

_____
_____
_____
_____

The guidelines and principles that I am today commissioning as my guiding principles and frames are— I understand that wealth is created by—

_____

___
___
___

The Intention Matrix
- Why become wealthy? What will wealth do for you?
- What's your magnificent obsession? Do you have a big enough *why* for all the challenges that wealth creation will bring?

My highest *intentions* in the back of my mind for becoming wealth are:

___
___
___
___

The Self Matrix
- Are you wealthy within yourself?
- Do you deserve to be wealthy?
- Do you see yourself as a wealthy or as a wealth creator?

The *meanings* that best enhance my identity as a wealth creator or as a wealthy person are—

___
___
___
___

The person I will become as a Wealth Creator is –

___
___
___
___

The Power Matrix
- What talents do you have or will develop to create wealth?
- What skills, passions, and interests will you use to add value to others or solve problems?
- What strategies do you have in place for creating wealth?

The actual wealth creation skills and strategies that I have, and will need to develop, are —

_____
_____
_____
_____

The strengths and weaknesses that I can play to as I develop my capacities of creating wealth are —

_____
_____
_____
_____

The Others Matrix
- Who will you work with and be on your team?
- Who will you collaborate with? Who will hold you accountable?
- What skills do you have for working with and through others?

The *relationships* that I have, and will build, with colleagues, clients, and customers, etc. include —

_____
_____
_____
_____

The interpersonal and social states, skills, and beliefs that will empower me for this are—

_____
_____
_____
_____

The States Matrix
- What are your top 10 wealth creation states?
- How wealthy are you in mind-and-emotion? In attitude?
- Have you tamed all your dragons and internal interferences that could sabotage you?

Inside-Out Wealth   *Chapter 15*   Your Wealth Creation Plan

The best *states* for accessing my best states and doing so persistently are —

_____
_____
_____
_____

Summary of my Empowering Decisions:
The empowering decisions that I am making today are —
The one thing I can do today to begin my wealth creation process is —

Examples:
 I will thoroughly learn this material by studying one chapter daily.
 I will begin to fill out my Wealth Creation Business Plan.

Summary of my Steps and Stages for my Ten Year Plan
The specific steps I will do in my wealth creation plan are the following:

_____
_____
_____
_____
_____
_____
_____
_____
_____
_____
_____
_____
_____
_____
_____
_____
_____
_____
_____
_____
_____
_____
_____
_____
_____
_____
_____
_____
_____
_____

Inside-Out Wealth   Chapter 15   Your Wealth Creation Plan

Meta-stating Wealth Creation

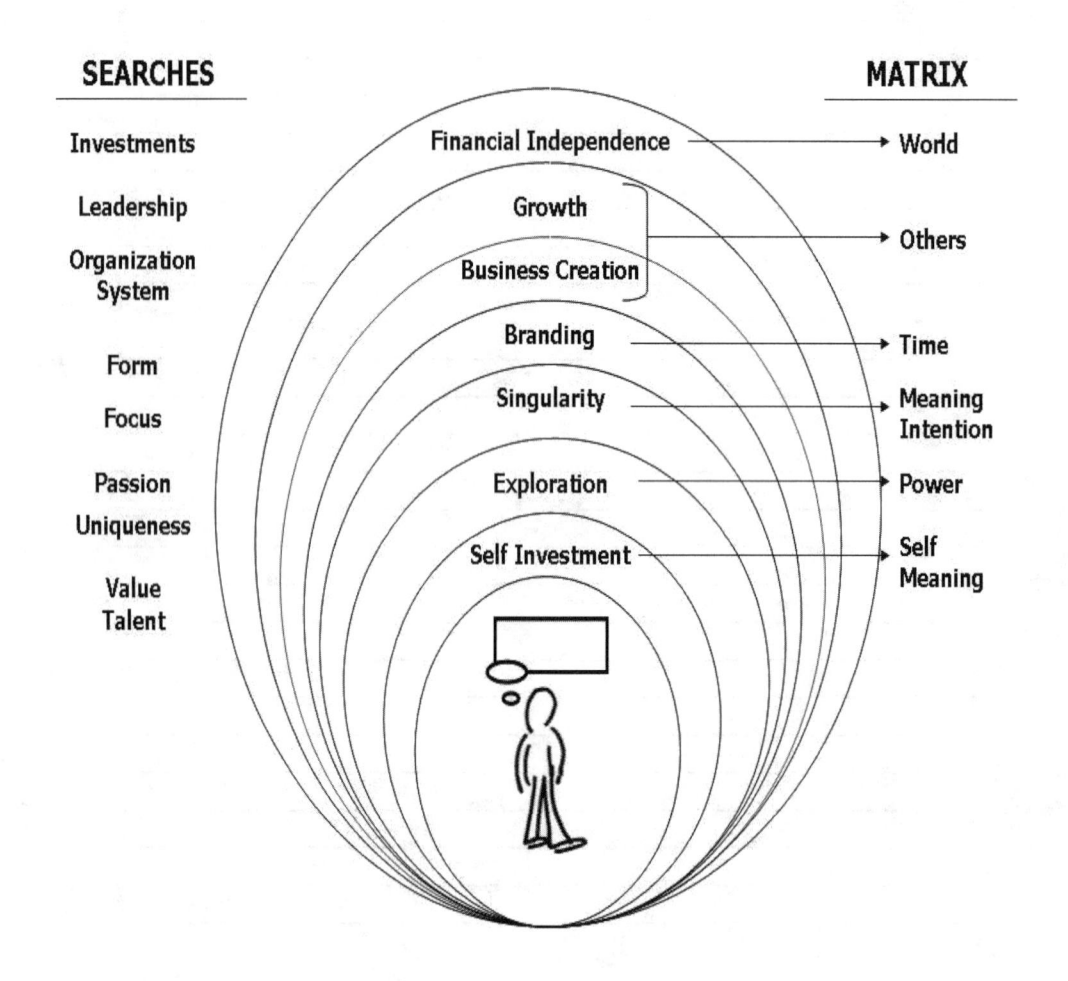

SEARCHES

Investments
Leadership
Organization System

Form
Focus

Passion
Uniqueness

Value
Talent

MATRIX

Financial Independence → World
Growth
Business Creation → Others
Branding → Time
Singularity → Meaning / Intention
Exploration → Power
Self Investment → Self Meaning

APPENDICES

Appendix A
Towards Defining Wealth

TIME-BINDING WEALTH

"Birds have wings— they fly. Animals have feet—they run. Man has the capacity of time-binding—he binds time." (Korzbyski, 1921, p. 145)

"We are a time-binding class of life." That was Alfred Korzybski's big discovery and his main point as he sought to create a solid foundation for his massive work, *Science and Sanity.* For Korzbyski time-binding was not a minor or sub-point in his work. Yet that's how I had always thought of it. So if you read some of my paragraphs in earlier books, that's how I presented time-binding. I treated it as a concept, an important one, but just as a sub-point in General Semantics. I was wrong.

Korzbyski himself actually said that Time-Binding Theory was the basis of all of his work and developments. What is this theory? *It is that our nature is to bind into ourselves*—into our minds and emotions, into our speech and actions, into our relationships to each other and to the world—*developments from earlier times.* While we are more than just that, this time-binding capacity and time-binging energy lies at the heart of what makes us unique in our kind of life.

In his *levels of life,* Korzbyski distinguished plants as the chemistry-binding class of life and animals as the space-binding. We also have these dimensions in our nature. We also take into ourselves chemicals and have a chemistry nature in our nervous system and cells. Humorously we say, "You are what you eat," And there's a great deal of truth in that. We also have the next dimension of reality within our nature. Like animals, we also *bind space* into ourselves. That's what makes environment, territory, context, movement, action, etc. so important in our way of life.

Yet in terms of dimensionality, we have yet another dimension to our being and nature that no other creature has—*time-binding.* This is the basis for our *ongoing progress*. This is why there's no need for us to reinvent the wheel, farming, industry, the steam engine, computers, the internet, etc. Why reinvent when you can adopt what others have invented and when you can improve it? This is the basis for being able to "stand on the shoulders of the giants" who have preceded us and to go beyond where they went in their discoveries.

The theory of time-binding explains lots of things about the unique human dimension of our lives. It positions language and symbolism as our central tools. After all, to bind into your nervous system and brain the learnings Aristotle made, you have to have *a way to transfer* what he knew inside to your insides. It isn't transferred by DNA. It isn't genetic. It is transferred by learning—by encoding your learnings in language, symbolism, diagrams, books, trainings, etc. so that others can bind the learnings into their mind and nervous system. No wonder it is so important to have an accurate or appropriate language system. If you map it inaccurately and falsely, the learnings will not transfer to create intellectual capital for you.

Ah, intellectual capital—this introduces another idea from Korzbyski, the idea of wealth-binding. While this is my phrase, the idea comes from Korzybski.
> "Civilization as a process is the process of binding time; progress is made by the fact that each generation adds to the material and spiritual wealth which it inherits." (106)

"The material and spiritual wealth" that we inherit! Wealth is not money. Wealth is the use of your time-binding powers as you use your brain to learn, figure out things, and invent ways of producing models, tools, processes, and cultures. These things comprise true "wealth"— intellectual capital.

Korzybski said that "wealth is production" (p. 80). From raw materials we produce tools and machines through our time-binding capacities of learning how to innovate our creations. Even raw materials, in and of themselves, are not wealth. It is not wealth to those who do not understand the raw materials, know what they are, how to use them, how to invent technology to deploy iron, oil, water, etc.

For that it takes intellectual wealth—it takes *time-binding energy*. This is the "energy" to learn—to learn from those who have gone before is a "higher energy," a mental or spiritual power, that you have by which you use your time-binding power to make past achievements live in the present and present activities in time-to-come. (p. 89). And because of this, *time* enters as an exponent in human progress.

Korzybski used the formula of **PT**^{t} to describe this time-binding power of progress and creativity. (**P** is for Progress, **R** for Rate and ^{t} for Time). The theory of time-binding in this mathematical formula says that *progress is a function of the rate that we can bind time.*

> "He becomes a civilized man only by the accumulation of dead men's work. Then and only then can he start where the preceding generation left off." (p. 123)

Ideally, human civilization could progress at an exponential rate. And in the hard sciences, we generally see things progress almost at that rate. With each generation, the new generation can accelerate growth and progress as we now see in the acceleration of change in our modern world with how quickly the newest inventions become obsolete and are replaced by the next generation.

What is wealth? Wealth is the time-binding power that gives you resources as "capital" that you can then build on.

> "Nature made man an increasing exponential function of time, a time-binder, a power that transforms and directs our basic powers." (129)
>
> "In nature's economy the time-binders are the intelligent forces. We are living in a world of wealth, a world enriched by many generations of dead men's toil." (131)
>
> "Animals do not produce wealth. Wealth consists of the fruits or products of this time-binding capacity. Human achievements and progress are cumulative knocking out the barriers of time. ... Wealth is almost entirely the product of the labor of by-gone generations."
>
> "Our wealth, civilization, everything we use and enjoy is in the main the product of the labor of men now dead. The wealth of the world is in the main the free gift of the past."

Wealth is knowledge—the ability to know, to learn, to connect things, to create models, to solve problems, and to add value. Wealth is the mind-and-heart of human beings understanding, caring, and making a difference. And we create all of this wealth as a "definitive mark of humanity." This is our "power to roll up continuously the ever-increasing achievements of generation after generation endlessly." (p. 110)

I really like one phrase Korzybski used in his description: "The living powers of the dead." If you think that sounds like the title of a horror movie, it is not. This phrase identifies that almost all of our wealth, all of the wealth on this planet, we did not create it in this generation. We inherited it from those who have preceded us. It is now *the living powers of the dead.* We inherit "the material and spiritual fruit of dead men's toil" which we can then augment in the brief span of our own lives, and then transmit it to our posterity. This is the process of civilization and shows that civilization itself is one of the things we create with our time-binding powers.

Appendix B
Playing the Wealth Creation Game

SEVEN PARADOXES OF WEALTH CREATION

To think like a millionaire, you may have to radically alter your current assumptions, beliefs, ideas, and even values. The more you operate from an inaccurate or impoverished map about *how to create wealth in the real world*, the more these principles will seem paradoxical, contradictory, non-sensical, and even counter-intuitive. Lots of things will be different:
- Your focus will be different
- Your sense of time and timing
- Your understanding of what wealth really is
- Your trust in luck versus taking personal responsibility
- Your experience and understanding of using frugality
- Your expectations of the process being easy or difficulty
- The focus of your investments

#1 THE FOCUS OF THE GAME:
Focusing on money prevents it; focusing on your passions invites money.
To play *the Wealth Creation Game,* find and develop your passion, the money will follow. As you get money out of your eyes, replace it with your loves. The more serious you are about money, the less effective you'll be. The more playful your relationship to money, the more likely you'll win the game.

The way to wealth is through absorption in your passion. It lies in the pathway of finding and following your passion, structuring your life around that passion, educating yourself in it, and giving yourself to it. Shape your work, associations, environment so that you can become more absorbed in it.

The way *not* to wealth is by focusing exclusively on money. A money-mindset prevents everything else from falling into place. So shift from making money your goal, defocus on it. Focus on doing what you enjoy and love and the money will follow. The paradox is that wealth is not really about money!

Harding Lawrence, CEO Chairman and CEO of Braniff
"Don't set compensation as a goal. Find work you like, and the compensation will follow. ... If money is a large part of your thinking, you won't do really good work, and that's what matters most. ... To me ... this was the field I loved. It wasn't a vocation. It was an avocation. I couldn't wait to get to work in the morning." (Blotnick, p. 52)

Too much interest in money actually interferes substantially with your efforts to become wealthy. It induces you into the wrong states (e.g. impatience, greed, snobbery, putting on airs, etc.). Set your wealth goals on doing something significant that adds value to others. Focus on something that's suited to your talents and interests, something you can easily invest all of your heart and soul into.

Enjoyment in the work itself will lead you to the right states (e.g., commitment, engrossing and deep satisfaction, creativity, exploration). It also leads you to developing skill and expertise. It reduces stress, the irritation with details, the undignified parts. It leads to greater involvement and focus. It changes the quality of the work, from "hard" work to absorbed work, from "job" to "mission."

Blotnick says that there is a "Millionaire's Lie" that many repeat so often that they actually come to believe it. The lie: "Creating wealth is all work, and no fun." Blotnick says this is just a way of defusing the fear that they are somehow "getting away with something" when they make a lot of money from doing something that they find engaging and a lot of fun.

#2   **THE SPEED OF THE GAME:**
The quickest route to getting rich is the slow route of patience.
As you play the Wealth Creation Game, if you operate from the "get rich quick" mind set, this will set you up for get rich quick schemes. Then you will be set up to be played by those who use deception to make you a sucker for their schemes. The quicker you get out of that state of mind, the quicker you can get on to the true pathway to wealth creation. Refuse that mentality. Decide to think long-term. Set your aim to play, *"Wealth in a decade."*

The more you want to be rich, the more impatient you'll become thereby lessening your likelihood of becoming rich. The more patience you access— the more likely you'll get there.

#3 **THE CONTENT OF THE GAME:**
The game of wealth is not about money; it is about internal abundance.
Wealth is first a wealthy mind—the wealth of ideas, values, and visions you care about. It's a mind-heart wealth that involves seeing and creating a solution to problems or hurts. Ideas that contribute and add value create wealth. "What value can I add? How can I contribute? How is this valuable? In what way? To whom? How can I use this to enhance my life? The life of others?"

The Game of Wealth Creation is really about becoming rich in all of the things that really count—mind, creativity, body, health, spirit, attitude, relationships, etc. When you have that, the finances will typically follow. The rule of the game then is to aim first and foremost to become rich in your mind and heart. Money is not about happiness, fulfillment, self-esteem, personal achievement, etc. There is only a two percent difference in *the happiness scale* between the wealthy and all other financial classes (Dent, 1998, p. 22).

Use money in your wealth creation process as a way to keep score of your financial success that will put you in a place of financial independence. Be aware of the problems that arise from over-valuing money. Suze Orman says, "People first, money second, things last." (First Law of Money, p. 50). Dent (*Roaring 2000s*) writes:
> "Surveys of happiness—wealth only affects the sense of well-being by a factor of Two percent. Happiness is more about relationships, friends, family, community, a balanced life. It's what you do with your life that counts. Wealth can be a tool for achieving the freedom to maximize your experience." (p. 22)

Reduce the meaning load on "money" so it doesn't mean too much. De-pleasure it so that it just "a means of exchange" and "a tool" for greater opportunities. Then it will not have you, *you will have it*. This will reduce its "demon hold" on you, its insatiable appetite for more, its arrogance that uses money as making your superior to others! Refuse money from becoming a dragon to you. "Ah, without it, I would feel insecure and inadequate. Without it, who would I be?"

#4 THE LUCK OF THE GAME:
The best luck comes when you don't depend on luck.
The more you trust "luck," the big deal, the quick buck, the more you lessen your chances for winning at the Wealth Game. The more responsibility you assume for your destiny, the more you increase your chances for winning. Shift your thinking from luck to response-ability, ownership, intelligent risk taking, proactive initiative, and efficiency.

The highest luck arises from taking complete ownership over what you think, do, act, relate, etc. Doing so improves your chances for creating wealth through saving, earning, investing, etc. Conversely, making excuses and blaming circumstance or person, the more you corrode your "luck" to win the game. It takes lots of courage to become wealthy; it also takes a game-like attitude. That is, an attitude that recognizes that it is just a game.

Robert Allen recommends replacing "luck" thinking with probability thinking.
> "I don't doubt there is such a thing as luck. But most of us give luck far too much credit. I don't think much about luck anymore, I pretend that it doesn't exit. I would rather look upon luck, as a low or a high probability of success." (p. 27)

#5 THE GAME OF SPENDING:
You pave the pathway to abundance on the street of frugality.
If wealth is not about money, then you cannot "spend your way to wealth." It doesn't work that way. Research has demonstrated again and again, that trying to "keep up" with the pace-setters, trying to "look the part," trying to drive the newest model of car, wear the most "in" clothes, surround yourself with all the status symbols of the "Rich and Famous" paradoxically, is the fastest way to debt and poverty. (*The Millionaire Next Door*; *The Millionaire Mind*).

More people who *look* wealthy on the outside are up to their necks in debt than the majority of the self-made millionaires who "live next door," shop at Sears, and drive a three-year old car. Don't fall for the toxic thought that "Looking, acting, and living a lifestyle of wealth attracts it." That superstition will not serve you well. It will lead you to a "paycheck to paycheck" living style. It leads to a pretend lifestyle of consumption, focusing on externals, seeking approval from others, etc.

The spending in the Game of Wealth that works is *spending your talents, passion, care, spending to develop yourself.* It is spending your attitude of appreciation so that you can use frugality to squeeze all the joy out of the stuff you have, etc.

#6 THE EASE OF THE GAME:
The easy way to win the wealth game is the tough path of self-mastery, personal independence, and mastery of a passion.
How easy or hard is it to become financially independent? Like mastery in any game, if you are always looking for the "easy and simple" way, the "get rich quick" schemes, then you will undermine your personal mastery of the game. You will stop yourself from developing the best wealth creation states (i.e., discipline, mastery, learning, patience, etc.).

The game is easy when you focus on truly mastering your passion, and becoming highly skilled as an expert at what you do. Then you will have loads of fun along the way. The way to enjoy any game is to have fun playing. Then it becomes a "flow" experience. Develop the strength to not sell out on your vision.

#7 THE INVESTMENT OF THE GAME:
The best investment payoff in the wealth game is to invest in yourself—in your skills, learning, and ongoing development.
In the 1980s Blotnick said that if you only have $50,000 to invest, then by all means invest in yourself, in your education, and in your skills. The best way to really invest in the Game of Wealth Creation is to focus on the source of true wealth. It comes from intelligence and creativity. It comes from men and

women with a passion to *contribute value* to something. They see a problem, a hurt, a need, and they set out to create a solution. True wealth arises in the mind of a person with vision, compassion, passion, and commitment. It arises from seeing and seizing opportunities. It consists of an attitude of focus on investing yourself, solving problems, determined persistence to keep at it, resilience to bounce back from any and every set back, human warmth and love.

Play the game by investing in continual self-education, in developing your imagination, creativity, problem solving skills, flexibility, expanding your sense of options, etc. If "An untrained mind cannot but help to create poverty," then conversely, a trained mind cannot but help see and seize opportunities for abundance.

Invest in your emotional intelligence also. Emotional intelligence is what allows you to effectively handle your positive and negative emotions so that you don't suffer in the poverty of self-pity, resignation, depression, anger-turned-into resentment, fear, etc. Invest in the emotional intelligence of state and meta-state management. The self-made millionaires of Stanley's study sorted for differences and were comfortable with thinking differently. That allowed them to see new things.

Appendix C
The Categories You Use for Money

BEWARE OF THE STRANGE WORLD OF MENTAL ACCOUNTING

How you represent, reckon, and appraise "money" determines how you respond to it. If the meanings that you give money, the mental categories and accounts in which you stash away your thoughts about money, set the frames for how you relate to money and how money relates to you—then your mental accounting plays a highly significant role.

> "A dollar here, a dollar there; pretty soon we're talking about real money."
> Anonymous

In an excellent research book, Gary Belsky and Thomas Bilovich address this facet of the psychology of mental accounting of money. These authors make the point that in your mental money accounting. "All money is not the same." Their first chapter is entitled, "Not all Dollars are Created Equal." As I read, I began sorting out the different "accounts" that they mentioned and created the chart that follows at the end of this appendix.[1]

Do you treat some "money" as play money, fun money, gift money, etc. and then blow it in ways that you would not dare to do with "savings?" *What mental categories do you use in thinking and relating to money.* Are your mental categories useful, effective, and empowering?
      Do they serve you well?
      Do they undermine your ability to save?
      Do they enhance your skills in wealth accumulation to build up enough capital to invest and get money to work for you?

Your Category Establishes your Use
If you have a category of, "college money for the kids" and a personal policy to "never touch it," then that might serve as a very useful classification trick to get you to save. To examine your own mental money accounting, step back and notice how you talk about money and notice the different kinds of money that you have in your mental world.

Belsky and Gilovich write:
> "Another way mental accounting can cause trouble is the resultant tendency to treat dollars differently depending on the size of the particular mental account in which they are stashed, the size of the

transaction within which they are spent, or simply the amount of money in question." (p. 37)

Imagine this *scenario:*
> You go to buy a lamp that costs $100. While in the store, you discover that you can get the very same lamp 5 blocks away for $75. You can save $25. Would you do it?
>
> Suppose also that you go to buy dining room set that's going for $1775, but only five blocks away you can get it for $1750. Do you go there to save $25?
>
> If you'll drive five blocks to save $25 for the first, but not the second, then the culprit at work in this is your *mental accounting.* You are treating the dollars differently due to how you think about the size of your purchase. So, when is $25 not $25?

Your mental accounting frequently causes you to relax your normal cost-consciousness when you make small purchases. The costs somehow get lost among larger expenses. For example, their research found that the bigger amount of "found money" you have (bonus, tax refund, gift, etc.), the more you experience it as sacred, serious, and harder to spend. Yet this actually lowers your "spending rate." Your *spending rate* refers to the percentage of an incremental dollar that you spend rather than save. So if you receive a $100 tax refund, and spend $80 of it, then your spending rate is .80.

What difference does this make? Here's an example of how mental accounting seduces over-spending. Studies showed that those who receive a $400 bonus use it to justify all manner of purchases, and in the end they spent 4 to 5 times that amount ($1,600 to $2,000).

> Who said?
> "Money was never a big motivation for me, except as a way to keep score. The real excitement is playing the game."[2]

Each time the couple reasons that they had just receive the big bonus. So they spend it, and spend it, and spend it. The accounting in their mind was that it wasn't "savings," it wasn't "living expenses," it was "extra," or "fun money." So while they went on a shopping spree, emotionally it didn't seem like a shopping spree. Because each smaller decision to splurge was kept in a different mental account.

Credit cards are one of the scariest exhibits in the museum of mental accounting. Credit card dollars are cheapened because there is seemingly *no sense of loss* at the moment of purchase, at least not on a visceral level. Conversely, if you have $100 cash in your pocket and pay $50 for something, you experience the purchase as cutting your pocket money in half. But if you "charge" it, you don't experience the same loss of buying power that emptying your wallet does. The money you charge on plastic is actually more costly if you don't pay it off.

"Dollars assigned to some mental accounts are devalued, which leads us to spend more easily and more foolishly, particularly when dealing with small amounts of money. And when account for other monies as so sacred or special, then we become too conservative with it." (p. 42)

THE DIFFERENT KINDS OF MONEY

Categories for Classifying Money	View of Money	Emotions	Response Style
Serious $	Real	Security, Cautious Safe	Save, Play
Windfall $ Fun $	Discretionary	Fun, Play With	Spend, Gamble
Gift $	Not really Mine	Treat as sacred	Don't spend
Slush Fund $ Vacation $	For extras For indulgence	Spend	
Funny $	Not quite real Credit Card $ Plastic $	Playful, Childlike	
Borrowed $	Credit Not like paying cash	Free; "not mine"	Spend without thought
Emergency $	Saving for a rainy day		
Mad $	Exists to use up and waste		Reckless

End Notes
1. Belsky, Gary; Gilovich, Thomas. (1999). *Why smart people make big money mistakes— and how to correct them.* NY: Simon and Schuster.

Appendix D

MILLIONAIRE-MIND CHECKLIST

- Do you think like a millionaire?
- Are your frames comparable to how a self-made millionaire thinks and feels?
- What are the key ideas, beliefs, understandings, decisions, intentions, etc. that govern and dominate the mind of a first-generation rich millionaire?

Check **T** for true and **F** for false. The more T-scores, the more ready and robust your Matrix of frames for wealth creation. The more F-scores, the more specific areas to address in developing your own plan for *inside-out wealth*.

> "The last thing we want to hear is the plain simple fact that *the rich think differently* than the poor. They are programmed differently. They have different expectations with respect to money. They have a wealth mindset. It is as if there were a filter between you and your world— the filter of your mind."
> Robert Allen

1) Work

___ I find my work absolutely fascinating, absorbing, and involving.

___ I can't wait to get up in the morning and get to the tasks and challenges of the day.

___ I can't believe that I actually get paid for what I'm doing.

___ It's not really work, it's what I love doing; I'm willing to work hard for what I believe in.

___ I don't aim for balance, I aim to make my work fun, enjoyable, and so meaningful it gives me vitality.

___ I focus on maximizing the return on my efforts.

___ I work harder than most people.

___ My heart and soul is completely into what I do.

___ I absolutely love my career.

___ I outperform my competition.

___ Because passion for a career is often *not* love at first sight, I know how to learn to love my work.

___ My work enables me to fully use and develop my abilities and aptitudes.

___ I am *willing* to be compensated on the basis of performance, I *want* it that way.

___ Total out of 13

2) Self-Development:

___ I am always thinking about how to become more competent and better at what I do.

___ As a life-long learner I believe that the only way to stay on top is to keep learning.

___ My day-job doesn't stop me from following my passions.

___ I'm always working on taking my skills and knowledge to the new level, always reading and learning.
___ I love challenges and see them as opportunities for growing and developing as a person.
___ I work on getting rid of any and all negative roadblocks in my head that stop me from succeeding and being all I can be.

___ Total out of 6

3) Money

___ Wealth creation and success is not just about money, it's about making a difference and touching lives.
___ Wealth is not the basis of happiness, it's just a scorecard. There's many things more important than money.
___ The status and prestige of wealth is not my primary interest. I'm more interested in the value that I create.
___ Money is a resource that should not be squandered.
___ For me, there are no limits on the amount of income I can make.
___ I think about the benefits of financial independence and freedom almost everyday.
___ I live well below my means.
___ I am frugal in getting all the joy and pleasure out of the things I already have.
___ I have a budget and keep track of my finances.
___ Wealth is all around us. There are thousands upon thousands of ways to create it.
___ Every dollar counts. I examine my financials regularly (at least once a week).
___ I have little or no debt except for a home or investment properties.
___ I do not borrow for lifestyle choices or items.
___ I use a shopping list to stay focused and avoid impulsive spending.
___ I clip coupons and use them in making purchases.
___ When I have success in making money I am not seduced by the ecstasy of buying lots of new things.
___ When my income increases significantly during a year, I do not automatically assume that will be my new base but recognize that markets and economies rise and fall.

___ Total out of 17

4) Adding Value

___ I love solving problems and creating new solutions.
___ I love the products I produce and services I provide.
___ I am following my passions and always learning to make them more marketable.
___ Giving quality service, creating quality products is what brings wealth.
___ Wealth is not money, but thinking, caring, creating, solving problems, seizing opportunities.
___ I take pride and pleasure in standing behind and guaranteeing my work (products and services).
___ I love seeing people enjoy the products and services that I produce.
___ I am always thinking about how I can add value to things.

___ Total out of 8

5) Business

___ I view mistakes as inevitable and a source of learning. I learn and make adjustments as quickly as possible.

___ I consider everything negotiable, asking the right questions, and creating a win/win arrangements.
___ There's always a solution. Every problem has dozens of good solutions.
___ I take full responsibility *for* my career, for the things I do and the results I get.
___ I am a nicher in that I am zero-ing in on a specialized field. (189)
___ I have a niche that gives my wealth creation focus and direction. (35)
___ I have found a profitable niche for my economic engine.
___ I thrive in my niche as I fully express my talents and interests.
___ I love selling my ideas, products, and services.
___ I never pay asking or retail price, I always negotiate.
___ I am ready to walk away from a deal at any time.
___ I work to ensure that my clients and customers receive the very best deal for their dollar.
___ To increase the odds of financial independence, I own my own business.
___ I have developed a niche where there's little competition.
___ In running my business I'm cost conscious and control my expenses.
___ I always ask for a discount and resolve to not pay full price.
___ I have found ideal career for my unique talents and aptitudes.
___ If what I am doing now is not my ideal job, I will learn everything I can about myself, this particular industry, and keep searching until I do.
___ I have the ability to sell my ideas, dream, products, services, and game plan.
___ I win my customers one at a time by devotion to their needs.
                ___ Total out of 20

6) *Risk*
___ There's no success without risk. Taking risks is what makes it exciting.
___ There is no financial security, my security is in myself, in my wits and creativity.
___ My security is in my knowledge, ability to learn and to adjust to changes, and to enjoy life for what it is.
___ The most risky thing is to be an employee and work for others.
___ It's risky to *not* be self-employed.
___ I take action on my plans. I create action plans and take the initiative to act on them.
___ The benefits of financial independence greatly outweighs the risks.
___ I capitalize on opportunities by knowing my niche, doing my homework, and developing more courage.
___ I regularly nurture my courage and counter my fears.
___ The biggest risk of all would be to let someone else control my career.
___ I control and manage my fears by taking charge of my believing in myself.
___ I have created a stable center in my life (home, friends, faith, etc.).
___ Risk is buying a home in a neighborhood where things are not appreciating.
___ I have a well-designed plan for "managing risks."
___ I take well-planned calculated risks in my business on a regular basis.
___ I constantly counter fear with courage.
                ___ Total out of 16

7) *Rich resourceful states*
___ I have a steel resolve that empowers my *persistence* on my way to wealth.
___ I have a burning desire to become financially independent.
___ I don't care that much about what others think, even authorities and experts.
___ I make up my own mind and follow my own visions.

___ I accept frustration as part of the game and work on increasing my *frustration tolerance*.
___ I *question* everything and don't assume that I have to accept the hand that has been dealt me.
___ It takes a lot of *courage and creativity* to create wealth opportunities.
___ I want and deserve wealth. I have the right to go for the best and to share the wealth.
___ It's critical to stay *focused* and to refuse being distracted with too many projects.
___ The power to say *no* to good things enables me to say *yes* to the best.
___ I am dependable, as good as my word and promises.
___ People can count on me for being *punctual, dependable, and responsible*.
___ I believe in myself and my ability to learn, adjust, and grow (*self-efficacy*).
___ Total out of 13

8) Time
___ Accumulating wealth takes time; I don't look for some short-term bonanza, I'm in it for the long-term.
___ It's not the timing of the market, but one's time in the market.
___ It takes patience and accumulated interest over years that builds incredible wealth.
___ Time is money, I use lists to prioritize my time and am in control of my time.
___ I spend time strengthening relationships.
___ When purchasing, I think about the lifetime costs and benefits.
___ I use a shopping list to save time, money, and avoid impulse buying.
___ I take time to plan for ways to use my time more productively.
___ I plan to reduce my waste of time and energy.
___ Frugality is buying quality items and making them last.
___ I do things like re-upholster and refinish furniture to extend the life-cycle of things.
___ When selling, I decide on my time parameters so I never panic.
___ I have control over how I allocate my time.
___ Time is money so I don't do do-it-yourself projects unless its part of my enjoyment.
___ Total out of 14

9) Relationships
___ It's all about relationships, working with and through others.
___ I believe in being personable with everybody I work with and so I act.
___ No one can be successful by themselves, it's the relationships.
___ Getting the right people on board is critical, people smarter than me who compliments my skills.
___ I am able to make others feel comfortable in my presence very quickly.
___ I have my ego out of the way sufficiently to create alliances and to set up collaborative partnerships.
___ I mostly use a coaching style in my communications and negotiations.
___ I enjoy a good competition and can be highly competitive.
___ I have (or have had) one or more mentors who enriched my life.
___ I don't follow the crowd in my purchases, clothes, ideas, etc., I think in unconventional ways.
___ I have superior social skills for getting along with people.
___ I want to be well respected and work to protect my reputation for integrity.

___ I am able to ignore the criticism of detractors and not let it bother me.
___ I don't take criticism personally.
___ My partner and I are both unselfish, caring, forgiving, understanding, and patient.
___ My partner and I have a common interest in wealth building activities (i.e., budgeting, sharing financial goals, etc.)
                                                    ___ Total out of 16

10) *Lifestyle*
___ I can enjoy economic success without having to adopt a Spartan lifestyle.
___ I focus on a comfortable lifestyle, but not an extravagant lifestyle.
___ I am not tempted or seduced by consumerism.
___ My interest in wealth creation is not about social status or displaying wealth.
___ I believe in balancing economic success and developing an enjoyable lifestyle.
___ My lifestyle puts me in contact with lots of people who become clients, customers, suppliers, friends.
___ Many of the best things in life are very inexpensive or even free (e.g. trips to museums, sporting event with kids, dinner with friends).
___ I prefer buying a house in an older and more established neighborhood.
___ I am not self-indulgent in my lifestyle.
___ I don't have to spend a lot of money to enjoy myself.
___ I am moderate in consumption and live a disciplined life-style.
___ The activities I do in my spare time enhance my wealth and creation of wealth.
___ Being well-organized in all facets of life is important to me.
___ I live in a well established neighborhood in a well-constructed home and see my home as a significant part of my investment portfolio.
___ I operate an economically productive household via frugality, planning, extending life cycle, etc.
                                                    ___ Total out of 15

11) *Character*
___ Know the importance of integrity, I strive to be honest with all people.
___ My integrity begins at home; I don't lie at all to my loved ones.
___ People will invest in you if they believe that you are honest and hardworking.
___ I fully recognize my limitations and weaknesses and have an unique strategy for compensating.
___ I believe that wealth is created through hard work, tenacity, getting along with people and discernment.
___ I have several strong leadership qualities.
___ I am very well organized.
___ I am well disciplined and enjoy being so.
___ I have extraordinary drive and resolve.
___ I work hard at my primary vocation and enjoy my free time doing what I enjoy.
___ I have the resolve to fight for what I believe in.
___ I have all five of the foundation stones for financial success: integrity, discipline, social skills, a supportive spouse, and hard work.
                                                    ___ Total out of 12

12) *Thinking Patterns*
___ I focus my energies and resources on maximizing output and results.
___ What's on my mind is success and solutions, not failures and problems.
___ I focus on quality over what's new, better, improved, or cheaper.
___ When one door is closed, I don't get discouraged, I get creative.

___ I am a finisher in a society of starters.
___ While I don't gamble or believe in luck, the harder I work the luckier I become.
___ I work hard and study thoroughly to invest in what I know.
___ I question the norm, the status quo, and the labeling of authority figures.
___ I have a strong work ethic.
___ When it comes to what I believe in and want, I am a fighter.
___ I think differently from the crowd and do not go along with the crowd.
___ I think strategically about things from shopping, scheduling to investing.
___ I am very deliberate in shopping for a home and invest time and planning.
___ I thinking in terms of how to make things more efficient and productive.

___ Total out of 14

13) Health and Fitness
___ I exercise regularly to be physically fit and have lots of energy.
___ I have extraordinary energy that I devote to my work and passions.
___ I value regular exercise for the energy and discipline it gives me.
___ Sports helps me to build an athletic heart of determination and self-discipline for mental toughness.

___ Total out of 4

14) Investments
___ I study the investments I make and seek advice for making intelligent investments.
___ I am, or plan to be, my own boss and own my own business.
___ I invest primarily in what I can control, namely my own business.
___ I surround myself with smart people when making financial decisions (a CPA, attorney, investment advisor).
___ I know how to select and work with getting good advisers on my team.
___ I calculate the probabilities of success with every investment.
___ "Waste not, want not" is one of my personal mottos.
___ I refuse to buy a home in a very short time, I can patiently wait.
___ I use real estate as part of my investment plans.
___ When investing in the stock market, I diversify and use a "buy and hold" strategy.

___ Total out of 10

15) Experiences
___ I have experienced the humiliation of defeat, been labeled inferior, or told that I didn't have what it takes.
___ I refuse to take the negative evaluations of authority figures seriously.
___ Having been confronted with challenges that would defeat others, I refuse to accept defeat.
___ I have bounced back from numerous set-backs.
___ Getting a "no" no longer discourages me, in fact, it now *excites* me.
___ I now have the tenacity of a bulldog, (or I have graduated from Tenacity #101).
___ I will never allow adversity to defeat my spirit or rob me of hope.

___ Total out of 7

16) Entrepreneurship
___ I see opportunities all around me.
___ I am not put off by low status occupations (e.g., pawn shops, salvage yard, car washes, etc.).
___ I am always looking for problems to solve.

___ I know how to sniff out opportunities.
___ I watch for and study trends and markets especially those that effect my area.
___ I am always exploring what ideas in books, conversations, courses that can I use in my business?
___ I am not seduced by the glamorous, high status occupations or trophy homes.

                                                        ___ Total out of 7

Grand Total out of 200 _____

[For your percentage, divide your T-score by 200, T-score ÷ 200 = ___ %, for example, a score of 100 is 50%, 150 is 75% and 180 is 90%]

___ 1) Work
___ 2) Self-Development
___ 3) Money
___ 4) Adding Value
___ 5) Business
___ 6) Risk
___ 7) Rich Resourceful States
___ 8) Time
___ 9) Relationships
___ 10) Lifestyle
___ 11) Character
___ 12) Thinking Patterns
___ 13) Health and Fitness
___ 14) Investment
___ 15) Experiences
___ 16) Entrepreneurship

> Based upon questionnaires from 733 self-made first-generation rich millionaires by Thomas J. Stanley, Ph.D. recorded in *The Millionaire Mind* (2000).
>
> Of these 733 from 1001 questionnaires, they averaged a net worth of 9.2 million, annual realized income of $749,000, only 2% inherited all or any part of their homes or property.

BIBLIOGRAPHY

Allen, Robert G. (1983/ 1986). *Creating Wealth.* NY: Simon and Schuster

Allen, Robert G. (1991). *No money down in the 90s.* NY: Simon and Schuster

Arterburn, Stephen. (1995). *Winning at work without losing at love.* Nashville, TN: Thomas Nelson Publishers.

Bandler, Richard; and Grinder, John. (1975). *The structure of magic, Volume I: A book about language and therapy.* Palo Alto, CA: Science & Behavior Books.

Bandler, Richard and Grinder, John. (1976). *The structure of magic, Volume II.* Palo Alto, CA: Science & Behavior Books.

Bandler, Richard. (1985). *Using your brain for a change: Neuro-linguistic programming.* Moab, UT: Real People Press.

Bandler, Richard; LaValle, John. (1996). *Persuasion Engineering: Sales & Business, Language & Behavior.* Capitola, CA: Meta Publications.

Bateson, Gregory. (1972). *Steps to an ecology of mind.* New York: Ballatine.

Belsky, Gary; Gilovich, Thomas. (1999). *Why smart people make big money mistakes—and how to correct them.* New York: Simon and Schuster.

Blotnick, Srully. (1980). *Getting rich your own way.* NY: Doubleday & Company.

Blotnick, Srully. (1980). *Winning: The Psychology of Successful Investing.* New York: Viking.

Blotnick, Srully. (1987). *Ambitious Men: Their drives, dreams, and delusions.* New York: Viking.

Burton, Ed. (1999). *Bulletproof Asset Protection:* How to stop some scumbag and his gold digging lawyers from taking your hard earned assets away.

Clawson, George S. (1926). *The richest man in Babylon.* NY: Penguin Books, New American Library.

Clements, Jonathan. (1998). *25 myths you've got to avoid—If you want to manage your money right: The new rules for financial success.* NY: Simon and Schuster.

Conti, Peter; Finkel, David. (2000). *How to create multiple streams of income.* Lakewood. CO.

Dilts, Robert; Grinder, John; Bandler, Richard; DeLozier, Judith. (1980). *Neuro-linguistic programming, Volume I: The study of the structure of subjective experience.* Cupertino. CA.: Meta Publications.

Davis, Kevin. (1996). *Getting Into Your Customer's Head: 8 secret roles of selling your competitors don't know.* NY: Random House, Times Business.

Dent, Harry S. Jr. (1998). *The roaring 2000s: Building the wealth and lifestyle you desire in the greatest boon in history.* NY: Simon & Schuster. Editor: Dominick Anfuso

Dominguez, Joe; Robin, Vicki. (1992). *Your money or your life: Transforming your relationship with money and achieving Financial*

Independence. NY: Viking

Eker, Harv. (2005). *Secrets of the millionaire mind: Mastering the inner game of wealth.* NY: HarperBusiness.

English, Gary. (1998). *Phoenix without the ashes: Achieving organizational excellence through common sense management.* NY: St. Lucie Press.

Fisher, Mark. (1988). *The instant millionaire: A millionaire reveals how to achieve personal and financial success.* London: Hammond.

Gitomer, Jeffery (1998). *Customer Satisfaction is Worthless; Customer Loyalty is Priceless.* Austin TX: Bard Press.

Goodman, Robert. (1996). *Independently wealthy: How to build financial security in the new economic era.* NY: John Wiley & Sons, Inc.

Gross, T. Scott. (1998). *Outrageous! Unforgettable service... guilt-free selling.* NY: AMACOM, American Management Association.

Hall, Michael L. (2000). Meta-states: Self-reflexiveness. Clifton, CO. Neuro-Semantic Publications.

Hall, L. Michael (2000). *Dragon slaying: Dragons to princes.* Clifton, CO. Neuro-Semantic Publications.

Hall, L. Michael. (1999). *Secrets of personal mastery.* Wales, UK: Crown House Publications.

Hall. L. Michael. (1999). *Frame Games.* Clifton, CO. Neuro-Semantic Publications.

Hansen, Mark Victor; Allen, Robert. (2002). *The one minute millionaire.* London: Vermilion.

Hill, Napolean. (1960). *Think and grow rich.* Greenwich, CN: A Fawcett Crest Book.

Kiyosaki, Robert T.; Lechter, Sharon L. (1997). *Rich dad/ Poor dad. What the rich teach their kids about money—that the poor and middle class do not!* Paradise Valley, AZ: TechPress, Inc.

Kiyosaki, Robert T.; Lechter, Sharon L. (2000). *Rich dad's cashflow quadrant: Rich dad's guide to financial freedom.* NY; Warner Books.

Korzybski, Alfred. (1933/ 1994). *Science and sanity: An introduction to non-Aristotelian systems and general semantics,* (5th. ed.). Lakeville, CN: International Non-Aristotelian Library Publishing Co.

Lesonsky, Rieva; Stodder, Galye. (1998). *Young millionaires: Inspiring stores to ignite your entrepreneurial dreams.* Irvine, CA: Entrepreneur Media Inc.

Locke, Edwin A. (2000). *The prime movers: Traits of the great wealth creators.* NY: AMACOM: American Management Association.

Machtig, Brett; Behrends, Ryan D. (1997). *Wealth in a decade.* Chicago: Irwin: Professional Publishing.

Maital, Shlomo; Maital, Sharone. (1984). *Economic games people play.* NY: Basic Books, Inc.

Maslow, Abraham. (1954/ 1970). *Motivation and personality.* New York: Harper & Row, Publishers.

Massnick, Forler. (1997). *The customer is CEO: How to measure what your customers want— and make sure they get it.* NY: AMACOM: American Management

Association.

McBride, Tracy. (1997). *Frugal luxuries: Single pleasures to enhance your life and comfort your soul.* New York: Bantam Books.

McKnight, Steve. (2003). *O to 130 Properties in 3.5 Years.* Milton Qld. Australia: Wrightbooks.

O'Connor, Joseph; Prior, Robin. (1995). *Successful Selling With NLP: The Way Forward in the New Bazaar.* London: Thorsons.

Orman, Suzie. (1999. *The courage to be rich: Creating a life of material and spiritual abundance.* NY: Penguin Books.

Rather, Dan (1999). *Striking it rich.* TV News Magazine: *48 Hours.* NBC. Thursday, April 1, 1999.

Robbins, Anthony. (1986). *Unlimited power: The new science of personal achievement.* NY: Simon and Schuster.

Senge, Peter M. (1990). *The fifth discipline: The art & practice of the learning organization.* NY: Doubleday

Sharma, Robin, S. (1997). *The monk who sold his ferrari:* San Francisco, CA: Harper San Francisco.

Sinetar, Marsha. (1987). *Do what you love, the money will follow.* NY: Dell Publishing; Division of Bantam Doubleday Dell Publishing Group.

Stanley, Thomas J.; Danko, William D. (1996). *The millionaire next door: The surprising secrets of America's wealthy.* Atlanta, GA: Longstreet Press.

Stanley, Thomas J. (2004). *Millionaire women next door.* Kansas City: Andrews McMeel Publishing.

Stossel, John. *Greed.* ABC Television Special. March 11, 1999.

Tarkenton, Fran. (1997). *What losing taught me about winning.* New York: Simon & Schuster.

Thurow, Lester C. (1999). *Building Wealth.* New York: HarperCollins Publisher.

Tracy, Brian. (2000). *The 100 absolutely unbreakable laws of business success.* San Francisco: Berrett-Koehler Publishers, Inc.

Trump, Donald J.; McIver, Meredith. (2004). *Trump: Think like a billionaire.* New York: Random House.

Trump, Donald J.; Kioyosaki, Robert T. (2006). *Why we want you to be rich: Two men, one message.* New York: Rich Press.

Tzougros, Penelope. (2004). *Wealthy choices: The seven competencies of financial success.* New York: Wiley.

Washington, Booker T. (1901). *Up From Slavery*, New York: Doubleday, Page and Co.

Wilde, Stuart. (1998). *The trick to money is having some!* Carlsbad, CA. Hay House, Inc.

INDEX

Abundance: 219, 249
Accountability: 146
ADD: 45-46
Appreciation: 77-78, 90
Attitude: 49-50, 215, 221

Being-Doing-Having: 23, 77, 137 146
Beliefs: see *Meanings*
Business:
   Creating a business: 166-182 (chapter 10)
   Entrepreneur-ing: 21, 34-36, 167-171
   Business Detailing: 171-175

Cashflow Quadrants: see *Money*
Collaboration: 17, 33, 150-165 (chapter 9)
   Criteria for: 158-160
   Networking: 163
Competitive: 151-152
Communication: 155-156, 157
Confrontation: 156
Courage: 200-206
Creativity: 64, 142-143

Debt: 102-104
Defusing: 161-162
Decision: 50-51
Desire: 42-43, 45
Dream: 8-26 (chapter 1)

Economics 101: 94-101
   Adding value: 94-97, 215
Efficiency: 208-210
Emotions: 41, 185-186
Fear: 194
Financial stability: 9
Financial independence: 9, 35, 109
Flexibility: 143
Flow state: 15
Frames of mind: 3
Frugality: 108-111, 251
Genius State: 17
Get Rich Quick: 1-2, 15, 24-28, 249
Greed: 70, 194
Health: 65
Identity: 132-149 (chapter 8)
Income: 107-112
Inner Game: 2
Inside-out-Wealth pattern: 130-131

Overview: 3-5, 22-24
Stages: 15-16, 28-38
Time-Line: 31, 37
Impatience: 195
Intention: 45-48
   Pattern: 47-49
   Clean intentions: 52
Integrity: 144-146
Interest: 120, 124
Investment: 178-180
Irritation Index: 119

Job: 101, 115-116, 117-119
Joy: 65, 115, 117, 159
   Joyful states: 215-221 (chapter 13)
Learned Helplessness: 138
Learned Optimism: 138-140
Learning: 137, 140-144
   Thinking like a Millionaire: 144, 256-262
Love: 216-217
Luck: 250

Matrix Model: 29-30, 235-243 (chapter 15)
Meaning: 28, 58-73 (chapter 4), 74-91 (chapter 5)
   Beliefs about: 76-87, 90
   Changing Beliefs: 87-89
   Definition: 82-87
   Meaning/ Performance: 29, 79-83
   Psycho-Logical: 84
Meta-Detailing: 171-175
Meta-States: 12, 13-15, 49, 199-213 (chapter 12)
   Meta-stating: 189-190
   Meta-Questions: 91, 119, 196
Modeling: 2-3, 10-15, 22, 162-163
   Strategies—TOTE model: 13-14
Money: 25, 59-66 (chapter 4)
   Accumulated interest: 106
   Assets and Liabilities: 111-112
   Budget: 101, 105
   Cashflow Quadrants: 20-21, 97-100
   Categorizing: 253-255
   Debt: 102-104
   Getting started: 101-112

Income: 62, 106-108
Investments: 36-37
Mental Accounting: 253-255
Meta-Levels of money: 60
Millionaire Mind Checklist: 256-262
Money Limits: 69-70
Psychology of: 67-69
Saving: 62-63, 104, 105-107
Time-Line: 31
Motivation: 42-57 (chapter 3)
   Big enough *Why*: 41-45, 50
   Rah-Rah! Motivation: 5, 45, 57
Multiple Intelligence: 117, 130

Negativity: 195
Negotiating: 160-161
Neuro-Semantics: 2-3, 12
NLP: 11
   Nominalizations: 76
Opportunities: 167-171
Optimism: 138-140
Inside-Out Wealth:
   Overview: 3-5
Passion: 118-122, 248-249
   Finding your passion: 118
   Creating your passion: 118, 120
My Personal Story:
   Chapter 1: 9-10
   Chapter 2: 39-40
   Chapter 3: 56-57
   Chapter 4: 71-72
   Chapter 5: 89-90
   Chapter 6: 112-113
   Chapter 7: 128-130
   Chapter 8: 140
   Chapter 9: 163-164
   Chapter 10: 180-181
   Chapter 11: 196-197
   Chapter 12: 211-212
   Chapter 13: 220-221
   Chapter 14: 232-234

Paradoxes: 248-252
Patience: 16, 174

Patterns
   Intentionality: 47-49
   Well-Formed Belief Criteria: 87
   Belief Change Pattern: 87-89
   Building a Matrix: 120
   Core Optimism Pattern: 139-140
   Inside-Out Pattern: 146-147
   Bigger than a Problem: 136
   Seeing Opportunities Pattern: 169
   Seizing Opportunities: 170-171
   Detailing Business Success: 175-176
   Selling Exploration: 176-177
   Accessing Your Best States: 188-189
   Escaping an Old Sabotaging Matrix: 193, 195-196
   Building Courage Meta-State: 201-202
   Holding a Risky Conversation: 205-206
   Building the Persistence You Need: 208
   Building Efficiency: 209-210
   Mind-to-Muscle: 229-232
   Seven Steps for Becoming Playfully Rich: 214-219

Persistence: 16, 174, 206-209
Planning: 54-56, 235
Play: 213
Power: 66
Resilience: 13, 210-211
Risk Taking: 177-178
Saving: 105-107
Security: 21, 99, 106, 194, 201-205
Self:
   Self-esteem: 133-134
   Self-acceptance: 133, 134-135
   Self-confidence: 133, 135
   Self-efficacy: 133, 135-137
   Self-capitalization: 133, 137
   Self-optimism: 133, 137-140
   Self-investment: 133, 140-144
   Self-integrity: 133, 144-146
   Self-Discipline: 111, 127
Self-Actualization Quadrants: 79-82
Self-Organizing Attractor: 47, 84
Selling: 176-177
Semantic Loading: 68
Shaping: 217-218
Singularity: 37, 122-125
Snobbery: 172

States: Chapters 11-13
   Composition: 185-186
   Lists: 184-185, 187-188

Accessing: 186, 188-189
Anchoring: 189
Gestalt states: 192-193
Meta-States: see *Meta-States*
Sabotaging states: 193

Taxes: 178
Talent Search: 117, 118-127
   SWOT analysis: 121
Team spirit: 157-158
Time: (chapter 2)
   Time-Line: 31
Trust: 153, 154-155
Value: 75-76, 94-96, 108, 122
Vitality: 216-217

Wealth: 58-73 (chapter 4)
   Adventure: 26
   Neuro-Semantics of: 61-62
   Definition of: 61-66, 75-76
   Wealth Creation Plan: 237-242
Work: 214-215

Persons

Aesop: 27
Allen, Robert: 20, 21, 33, 64, 126, 127, 177, 178, 201, 250, 256
Anixter, Alan: 169
Arterburn, Stephen: 141

Bandler, Richard: 12, 85, 113
Bartlett, Ken: 55-56
Belsky, Gary: 253-255
Bilovich, Thomas: 253-255
Blotnick, Scrully: 14-19, 38, 52, 127, 142, 143, 153, 172, 174, 194, 249, 251
Brehends, Ryan: 37, 83, 93, 110
Bridoux, Denis: 98, 100

Carnegie, Dale: 207
Clawson, George: 126, 215
Clements, Jonathan: 27, 104
Collins, Jim: 25, 122
Cox, Collin: 197

Danko, William: 19, 65, 109, 110, 116, 126, 145, 168, 207, 208
David, George: 64
Dent, Harry: 36, 63, 204, 250
Dilts, Robert: 14, 84
Disney, Walt: 191
Disraeli, Benjamin: 42, 58

Dominquez: 61, 109
Drucker, Peter: 143
Dystel, Oscar: 52

Eker, Harv: 125, 150
Emereson, Ralph Waldo: 1, 115
Epictetus: 115
Feather, William: 206

Gardner, Howard: 130-131
Gibbson, Edward: 64
Grinder, John: 13

Harvey, Paul: 210
Hill, Napolean: 44, 51, 58, 74, 78, 142, 155, 191, 207
Kiyosaki, Robert: 19-20, 64, 69, 97-100, 125, 142, 146, 166, 178, 190, 194, 195, 199, 204, 210, 216
Korzybski, Alfred: 244-247
Lawrence, Harding: 248

MacArthur, Douglas: 201
Machtig, Brett: 37, 53, 63, 93, 104, 110, 208
Maslow: Abraham: 214
May, Rollo: 45
Mellan, Olivia: 67
Miller, George: 13

Orman, Suze: 23, 59, 93, 184, 199, 199, 250
O'Reilly, B.: 173
Porras, William: 25
Robbins, Anthony: 42, 54, 184, 219
Rohn, Jim: 144
Rockefeffer, John D.: 70
Schwab, Charles: 74
Seligman, Martin: 138
Senge, Peter: 42
Sinetar, Martha: 78, 116, 132, 133, 190
Stanley, Thomas: 19, 52, 62, 80, 109, 110, 116, 126, 143, 144, 145, 202, 204, 205, 207, 208, 217, 262
Stone, W. Clement: 206
Tracy, Brian: 150
Trump, Donald: 27, 65, 77, 111, 142, 172, 205, 213, 216
Turner, Ted: 70
Walters, Barbara: 70
Washington, Booker T.: 78
Williams, Paul: 142

L. Michael Hall, Ph.D.

Modeler of Excellence
Using Neuro-Semantics and Self-Actualization Psychology

L. Michael Hall is a visionary leader in the field of NLP and Neuro-Semantics, and a modeler of human excellence. Searching out areas of human excellence, he models the structure of that expertise and then turns that information into models, patterns, training manuals, and books. With his several businesses, Michael is also an entrepreneur and an international trainer.

His doctorate is in the Cognitive-Behavioral sciences from Union Institute University. For two decades he worked as a psychotherapist in Colorado. When he found NLP in 1986, he studied and then worked with Richard Bandler. Later when studying and modeling resilience, he developed the Meta-States Model (1994) that launched the field of Neuro-Semantics. He co-created the *International Society of Neuro-Semantics* (ISNS) with Dr. Bob Bodenhamer. Learning the structure of writing, he began writing and has written more than 40 books, many best sellers in the field of NLP.

Applying NLP to coaching, he created the Meta-Coach System, this was co-developed with Michelle Duval (2003-2007), he co-founded the Meta-Coach Foundation (2003), created the Self-Actualization Quadrants (2004) and launched the new Human Potential Movement (2005).

Wealth Biography
Growing up in mid-America in a middle-class home, Michael's father, Louis Joseph Hall, was a mathematics teacher at the local high school— the first in his family to go to University. But having grown up in the Depression Years in the US (1929-1940) inherited all the fears associated with poverty and the lack of understanding of how wealth is created.

So did Michael. Following his dad's example of working in a helping industry rather than pursuing a career in a high finance career, it wasn't until a financially-devastating divorce woke him up that he even thought about how to create wealth or its importance. So at 37 and the tools of a new discipline (NLP), he set out to avoid financial ruin. Another ten years passed, and having achieve financial stability, a new idea emerged— financial independence and freedom. The freedom to make decisions based on desire of what one wants to do rather than needs to do financially.

So at 46, he set out to model the structure of wealth creation. Eight years later he reached his first million, something that surprised him because he was not focusing on that. It essentially happened "when I wasn't looking."

The search for the process and secrets of wealth creation led to other surprises and forms of wealth—discovering new models in NLP, creation of hundreds of new patterns for personal effectiveness, founding a new field of self-actualization (Neuro-Semantics), founding a new world-class training for professional coaches (Meta-Coaching), the production of scores of books and training manuals, etc. And the abundance of this creative wealth then gave birth to a vision for Neuro-Semantics as an international community.

Dr. Hall often says that he began the modeling of wealth creation simply and solely to get out of debt, stop the creditors, get beyond living paycheck to paycheck. Later his goal shifted to having enough to make decisions about what to do *not* based on consulting his financial needs. Discovering that the models worked in his own life, he began teaching wealth creation as one of the training of Neuro-Semantics. He has now taught *Inside-Out Wealth* around theworld from New York to London, France, Moscow, Johannesburg, South Africa, Sydney to San Francisco.

Contact Information:
P.O. Box 8
Clifton, Colorado 81520 USA
(1-970) 523-7877

Websites:
www.neurosemantics.com
www.meta-coaching.org
www.self-actualizing.org
www.meta-coachfoundation.org

Books by L. Michael Hall, Ph.D.

1) *Meta-States: Mastering the Higher Levels of Mind* (1995/ 2000)
2) *Dragon Slaying: Dragons to Princes* (1996 / 2000)
3) *The Spirit of NLP: The Process, Meaning and Criteria for Mastering NLP* (1996)
4) *Languaging: The Linguistics of Psychotherapy* (1996)
5) *Becoming More Ferocious as a Presenter* (1996)
6) *Patterns For Renewing the Mind* (with Bodenhamer, 1997 /2006)
7) *Time-Lining: Advance Time-Line Processes* (with Bodenhamer, 1997)
8) *NLP: Going Meta — Advance Modeling Using Meta-Levels* (1997/2001)
9) *Figuring Out People: Reading People Using Meta-Programs* (with Bodenhamer, 1997, 2005)
10) *SourceBook of Magic, Volume I* (with Belnap, 1997)

11) *Mind-Lines: Lines For Changing Minds* (with Bodenhamer, 1997/ 2005)
12) *Communication Magic* (2001). Originally, *The Secrets of Magic* (1998).
13) *Meta-State Magic: Meta-State Journal* (1997-1999).
14) *When Sub-Modalities Go Meta* (with Bodenhamer, 1999, 2005). Originally entitled, *The Structure of Excellence.*
15) *Instant Relaxation* (with Lederer, 1999).
16) *User's Manual of the Brain: Volume I* (with Bodenhamer, 1999).
17) *The Structure of Personality:* Modeling Personality Using NLP and Neuro-Semantics (with Bodenhamer, Bolstad, and Harmblett, 2001).
18) *The Secrets of Personal Mastery* (2000).
19) *Frame Games: Persuasion Elegance* (2000).
20) *Games Fit and Slim People Play* (2001).

21) *Games for Mastering Fear* (with Bodenhamer, 2001).
22) *Games Business Experts Play* (2001).
23) *The Matrix Model: Neuro-Semantics and the Construction of Meaning* (2003).
24) *User's Manual of the Brain: Master Practitioner Course, Volume II* (2002).
25) *MovieMind: Directing Your Mental Cinemas* (2002).
26) *The Bateson Report* (2002).
27) *Make it So! Closing the Knowing-Doing Gap* (2002).
28) *Source Book of Magic, Volume II, Neuro-Semantic Patterns* (2003).
29) *Propulsion Systems* (2003).
30) *Games Great Lovers Play* (2004).

31) *Coaching Conversation, Meta-Coaching, Volume II* (with Duval, 2004).
32) *Coaching Change, Meta-Coaching, Volume I* (with Duval, 2004).
33) *Winning the Inner Game* (2006, formerly *Frame Games,* 1999).
34) *Unleashed: How to Unleash Potentials for Peak Performances* (2007).
35) *Achieving Peak Performance* (2009).
36) *Self-Actualization Psychology* (2008).
37) *Unleashing Leadership* (2009).